ILLUSTRATED SELF ASSESSMENT IN
PAEDIATRICS

Publisher: Richard Furn
Project Development Manager: Fiona Conn
Project Manager: Frances Affleck
Designer: Judith Wright

ILLUSTRATED SELF ASSESSMENT IN
PAEDIATRICS

Tom Lissauer

MB BChir FRCP FRCPCH
Consultant Paediatrician
St Mary's Hospital, London, UK

Graham Roberts

BM BCh MA MRCP MRCPCH
Research Fellow in Paediatric Allergy
St Mary's Hospital, London, UK

Caroline Foster

BA MBBS MRCP MRCPCH
Specialist Registrar in Paediatric Infectious Diseases
St Mary's Hospital, London, UK

Michael Coren

BSc MBBS MRCP MRCPCH
Consultant Paediatrician
St Mary's Hospital, London, UK

Illustrations by: MTG

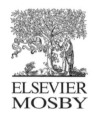

ELSEVIER
MOSBY

EDINBURGH LONDON NEW YORK OXFORD PHILADELPHIA ST LOUIS SYDNEY TORONTO 2001

MOSBY
An imprint of Elsevier Limited

First published 2001
   Reprinted 2004, 2005 (twice)

ISBN 0 7234 3177 9

British Library Cataloguing in Publication Data
A catalogue record for this book is available from the British Library

Library of Congress Cataloguing in Publication Data
A catalogue record for this book is available from the Library of Congress

Notice
Medical knowledge is constantly changing. As new information becomes available, changes in treatment, procedures, equipment and the use of drugs become necessary. The author, contributor and the publishers have, as far as it is possible, taken care to ensure that the information given in this text is accurate and up to date. However, readers are strongly advised to confirm that the information, especially with regard to drug usage, complies with the latest legislation and standards of practice.

ELSEVIER your source for books, journals and multimedia in the health sciences

www.elsevierhealth.com

Working together to grow
libraries in developing countries

www.elsevier.com | www.bookaid.org | www.sabre.org

ELSEVIER   BOOKAID International   Sabre Foundation

The
publisher's
policy is to use
**paper manufactured
from sustainable forests**

Printed in China
C/04

Contents

Preface

The aim of this book is to consolidate knowledge of paediatrics and aid revision for examinations. None of us likes exams but self assessment can be an important driving force for learning. This book accompanies the *Illustrated Textbook of Paediatrics* (2nd edition) by Tom Lissauer and Graham Clayden which contains all the core information on which the questions are based. It is primarily designed for medical students, but it is also suitable for candidates preparing for postgraduate paediatric examinations such as the Diploma of Child Health (DCH) and Membership of the Royal College of Paediatrics and Child Health (MRCPCH), although candidate for these latter examinations would be expected to score higher marks. Answers are provided for all the questions, often with additional comments or explanation.

We have used varied formats for the questions and answers. In addition to standard multiple choice questions, some of the questions are in the 'best of five' format, or involve selecting a number of items from a larger list, or are open-ended questions where appropriate. Throughout the text we have tried to minimise the amount of writing required, by using tables which simply need to be completed with ticks in the appropriate places, and by asking for clinical scenarios to be matched with the most likely diagnoses. We very much hope that the variety of content and format that we have included will make the book interesting as well as instructive.

While there is of necessity some testing of basic knowledge, we have also tried to test understanding and decision making. We have concentrated on the most important topics within paediatrics and have avoided rare problems unless an important message is conveyed.

We welcome feedback about the book.

Tom Lissauer
Graham Roberts
Caroline Foster
Michael Coren
2001

Acknowledgements for slides

The authors would like to thank the following people for contributing figures:

Dr Saad Abdalla fig 13.9
Dr Paula Bolton-Maggs fig. 20.1
Dr Graham Clayden fig. 25.7
Dr Jon Couriel figs 14.3 & 14.6
Dr Jane Deal fig. 16.4
Dr Tony Hulse fig 25.5
Dr Deirdre Kelly fig. 18.2
Dr Michael Markiewicz fig. 16.6
Dr Peter Reynolds fig. 8.3
Mr Neil Tolley figs 14.1 & 14.2
Professor Julian Verbov figs 22.2, 22.3, 22.4, 22.5, 22.7, 22.8 & 22.9b
Dr Jeremy Wales figs 10.5, 23.2 23.3, 23.4, 23.5, 24.3, 25.1, 25.2 &25.3

1 The child in society

1. *Complete the following table, comparing child health in developing and developed countries, by placing a tick in the appropriate box. For each question, neither, one or both boxes may be correct.*

		Developing countries	Developed countries
A	Children constitute a higher proportion of the population	✓	
B	The proportion of newborn babies who are of low birth weight (< 2.5 kg) is higher	✓	
C	The childhood mortality rate is declining more rapidly	✓	
D	The commonest cause of death in children is from road traffic accidents		✓
E	The immunisation uptake rate is higher		✓

1.

	Developing countries	Developed countries
A Children constitute a higher proportion of the population	✓	
B The proportion of newborn babies who are of low birth weight (< 2.5 kg) is higher	✓	
C The childhood mortality rate is declining more rapidly	✓	
D The commonest cause of death is from road traffic accidents		✓
E The immunisation uptake rate is higher		✓

A   As a country's gross national product increases, children constitute a smaller proportion of the population and the elderly a higher proportion.

B   The proportion of newborn babies who are of low birth weight (< 2.5 kg) is much higher in developing countries.

C   The childhood mortality rate in developing countries is much higher and is declining more rapidly. However, in some countries in sub-Saharan Africa, HIV infection has arrested the decline in mortality. In developed countries, childhood mortality is low and its further decline is slow.

D   Whereas the commonest cause of death in childhood in developed countries is from road traffic accidents, in developing countries it is the result of infectious diseases.

E   The overall immunisation uptake is higher in developed countries.

2 History and examination

1. *Alexander, aged 13 months, is brought by his mother to his general practitioner with a one-day history of vomiting and diarrhoea. He has not had any significant illnesses in the past. In taking the history:*

(handwritten: GASTROENTERITIS)

i) Concerning the vomiting, what two further features would you ask about?

ii) Concerning the diarrhoea, what two further features would you ask about?

iii) List two other questions you would ask. *(handwritten: • Travel / Contact / Fluid intake / fever, Rash, Pain, urine output iv))*

You diagnose mild gastroenteritis and advise glucose electrolyte mixture for 24 hours followed by a return to a normal diet.

iv) What specific advice would you give to his mother to ensure that she knows under what circumstances she should again seek medical attention for this illness? List three points. *(handwritten: signs of dehydration)*

2. *Which of the following statements about the clinical examination of a child are true or false:*

A Central cyanosis is best assessed by examining the nail beds

B Stridor is a low-pitched expiratory sound from distal airway obstruction *(handwritten: INSPIRATION)*

C A thrill at the left sternal edge may be caused by increased blood flow associated with a high fever *(handwritten: pulse; should heart lesion – serious)*

D The femoral pulses are reduced in patent ductus arteriosus *(handwritten: (Co-arctation of the aorta))*

E An enlarged spleen moves with respiration

(handwritten: Bounding Pulse)

3. *Jason, aged three years, has been febrile and short of breath for 24 hours.*

The findings on examination of his chest are shown in Fig. 2.1. Select the single most likely diagnosis from the list below:

A Asthma *(handwritten: (↑, wheeze on expiration))*

B Pneumonia

C Pneumothorax *(handwritten: (↓ movement))*

D Cardiac failure

E Pleural effusion *(handwritten: (Bilateral))*

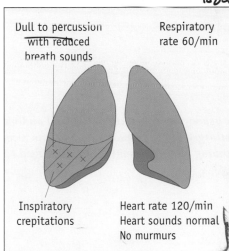

Dull to percussion with reduced breath sounds

Respiratory rate 60/min

Inspiratory crepitations

Heart rate 120/min
Heart sounds normal
No murmurs

Fig. 2.1 *(handwritten: PNEUMONIA.)*

Answers (right margin, handwritten)

1. i) Volume, Colour, Any Blood

ii) Blood, Mucus, How much?, Consistency

iii) ? Abdominal Pain, ? First illness

2.
A True ☐ False ☑
B True ☐ False ☑
C True ☑ False ☐
D True ☐ False ☑
E True ☑ False ☐

3. A B C D E

4. *Ritha, aged 10 months, is admitted to hospital with a two-day history of mild coryza and difficulty breathing.*

i) Place a tick in the table to show which clinical features suggest respiratory or cardiac disease. Some features may apply to both.

		Respiratory	Cardiac
A	Failure to thrive	✓	✓
B	Poor feeding	✓	✓
C	Sweating		✓
D	Generalised wheeze on auscultation	✓	✓
E	Marked hepatomegaly	✗	✓

4. ii)

← Generalised wheeze on auscultation,

ii) List three clinical features which would indicate that Ritha's respiratory distress is severe. Nasal flaring, Tachypnoea, intercostal recession, tracheal tug, Diaphragmatic Tug, Harrison's sulcus

→ Displaced by HYPERINFLATION

5. *Match the following histories with the diagnoses listed in the table:*

5. BRONCHIOLITIS, BUT IT IS NOT ENLARGED

A A mother has noted that her 14-month-old son's abdomen appears to be swollen. He is well and has no bowel or urinary symptoms. The general practitioner feels a large mass on the left side of the abdomen which does not cross the midline.

B A 15-month old boy presents with episodes of abdominal pain over the previous 12 hours. He has vomited twice. On examination he is unwell and poorly perfused. There is a mass in the right upper quadrant of his abdomen.

C A 13-year old girl has been unwell for a few weeks with fever, anorexia and a sore throat. On examination there is 3 cm splenomegaly. A full blood count shows atypical lymphocytes.

DIAGNOSES

Case histories	Intussusception	Neuroblastoma	Leukaemia	Infectious mononucleosis	Wilms' tumour
A					✓
B	✓				
C				✓	

6. *Nazma, aged four years, presents with pallor and abdominal pain. On examination an enlarged spleen is palpable. She has recently arrived from Kenya. Which of the following might account for her enlarged spleen?*

A Acute lymphoblastic leukaemia

B Malaria

C Thalassaemia

D Hookworm infestation

E Coeliac disease

6.

A True ☐ False ☐
B True ☐ False ☐
C True ☐ False ☐
D True ☐ False ☐
E True ☐ False ☐

7. *Which of the following statements about the neurological examination of a child are true or false:*

A   Unilateral walking on tiptoe in an 18-month-old is a feature of hemiplegia

B   Scissoring of the legs on lifting a nine-month-old infant under the arms is a feature of cerebral palsy

C   Nystagmus is a normal variant in toddlers

D   Increased limb reflexes and ankle clonus are a feature of lower motor neurone lesions

E   Hand preference in an eight-month-old is a normal variant

8. *Katie, aged 18 months, is still very unsteady on her feet. She tends to fall to her left side. Her limb tone and reflexes are shown in Fig. 2.2.*

i) Select the site of the neurological lesion:

    A   Upper motor neurone lesion

    B   Lower motor neurone lesion

    C   Cerebellar lesion

    D   Basal ganglia lesion

    E   Neuromuscular junction

ii) Which of the following best describes the pattern of neurological signs:

    A   Diplegia

    B   Right hemiplegia

    C   Left hemiplegia

    D   Spastic quadriplegia

    E   Choreoathetoid cerebral palsy

7.

A   True ❑   False ❑
B   True ❑   False ❑
C   True ❑   False ❑
D   True ❑   False ❑
E   True ❑   False ❑

8. i) A B C D E
    ii) A B C D E

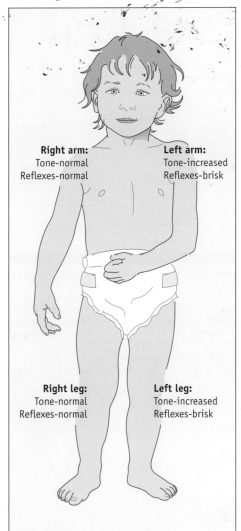

Right arm:
Tone-normal
Reflexes-normal

Left arm:
Tone-increased
Reflexes-brisk

Right leg:
Tone-normal
Reflexes-normal

Left leg:
Tone-increased
Reflexes-brisk

Fig. 2.2

9. *Seb, aged six years, has recently returned to the UK from visiting his relatives in Thailand. Over the last few weeks his mother has noticed a large gland in his neck.*

   i) List two possible non-malignant causes.

   ii) Give two features that would suggest a malignant cause on examination of the gland or on general examination.

10. *Sally, aged eight years, complains of recurrent headaches. Her blood pressure is measured as 140/90. Give one reason why this might be erroneously high.*

9. i)

   ii)

10.

1. i) Bile staining of vomit
       Presence of blood or altered blood in vomit
       Frequency/severity of vomiting
   ii) Blood/mucus in stool
       Frequency/severity of diarrhoea
   iii) Contact with other affected people
       Travel
       Fluid intake
       Associated features e.g. fever, rash, pain, urine output
   iv) Failure to tolerate oral fluids
       Vomiting/diarrhoea gets worse
       Bile appears in vomit
       Blood appears in vomit/diarrhoea
       Reduced urine output – fewer wet nappies
       Becomes drowsy or overall condition deteriorates
       Parents are worried

[handwritten: BILE / BLOOD / FREQ severity vomiting]
[handwritten: BLOOD/MUCUS STOOL FREQ/SEVERITY DIARRHOEA]
[handwritten: Blood / Bile in vomit worse. Failure to tolerate ORAL FLUIDS Reduced urine o/p – fewer wet nappies. becomes drowsy or overall condition deteriorates. Parents are worried]

2. A *False.* It is best assessed on the tongue.
   B *False.* It is a low-pitched inspiratory sound from upper airway obstruction.
   C *False.* A thrill is a palpable murmur caused by a turbulent flow of blood from structural heart lesion.
   D *False.* With a patent ductus arteriosus (PDA) the femoral pulses are bounding; they are reduced with coarctation of the aorta. → *[handwritten: Pulse is bounding]*
   E *True.*

3. B *[handwritten: PNEUMONIA.]*

4. (i)

		Respiratory	Cardiac
A	Failure to thrive	✓	✓
B	Poor feeding	✓	✓
C	Sweating		✓
D	Generalised wheeze on auscultation	✓	✓
E	Marked hepatomegaly	*	✓

*The liver may be displaced downwards by chest hyperinflation in bronchiolitis, but is not enlarged

   ii) Signs of increased respiratory effort:
       ● marked tachypnoea, nasal flaring, grunting on expiration, marked intercostal/subcostal recession
       Signs of hypoxaemia:
       ● marked tachycardia, agitation, drowsiness, cyanosis

[handwritten: (Tachycardia, cyanosis + agitation + drowsiness)]

5.
DIAGNOSES

Case histories	Intussusception	Neuroblastoma	Leukaemia	Infectious mononucleosis	Wilms' tumour
A					✓
B	✓				
C				✓	

6. A *True.*
   B *True.*
   C *True.* Thalassaemia may occur in children of Asian origin. Presenting at three years of age, it would be more likely to be thalassaemia intermedia than thalassaemia major.
   D *False.*
   E *False.*

7. **A**   *True.* This is because of increased muscle tone leading to a tight Achilles tendon.
    B   *True.* This is due to increased adductor tone in the legs.
    C   *False.*
    D   *False.* These are features of an upper motor neurone lesion.
    E   *False.* Hand preference is abnormal below one year of age.

8. i)   **A**
    ii) **C**

9. (i)   Reactive lymphadenopathy from upper respiratory tract infection
          Infected lymph node
          Dental abscess
          Infectious mononucleosis
          TB
          Atypical mycobacterial infection
    ii)   Gland large and rubbery
          Non-tender
          Tethering to underlying tissues
          Associated signs:
              anaemia
              bruising
              petechiae
              hepatosplenomegaly
              enlarged glands at other sites

10. If the blood pressure cuff is too narrow ($< \frac{2}{3}$ of the upper arm length), or if she is upset or in pain.

3 Child development, hearing and vision

1. *Complete the table of normal developmental milestones by placing a tick in the corresponding box.*

Developmental milestones	Median age			
	6 weeks	3 months	6 months	12 months
A Sits unsupported				
B Reaches for objects				
C Smiles responsively				
D Says one or two single words with meaning				
E Walks unsupported				

2. *At an 8-week surveillance review you would expect an infant to:*

A Roll over

B Quieten to certain sounds

C Fix and follow a moving face

D Grasp an object placed in his hand

E Say 'dada' without meaning

2.

A True ❏ False ❏

B True ❏ False ❏

C True ❏ False ❏

D True ❏ False ❏

E True ❏ False ❏

3. *A health visitor refers Graham, aged nine months, for further assessment. He was born at term and has had no medical problems. His mother now reports that he can roll over but cannot sit unsupported. He is vocalising 'mamma' and 'dada'. The health visitor notices that when playing he reaches for objects predominantly with his left hand.*

i) Other than delayed sitting, what developmental feature of concern has the health visitor identified?

ii) What is the most likely diagnosis?

3. i)

    ii)

4. *Would you expect a one-year-old girl to:*

A Scribble with a pencil

B Reach for a small object with a good pincer grip

C Finger feed and drink from a feeding cup

D Build a tower of three bricks

E Be able to remove her T-shirt

4.

A True ❏ False ❏

B True ❏ False ❏

C True ❏ False ❏

D True ❏ False ❏

E True ❏ False ❏

5. *India, aged 12 months, is assessed by her general practitioner because she is not yet crawling. She can roll over and sit without support. She can get across the floor to reach objects but does this in the sitting position using her legs to push herself along the floor. She is able to stand while holding on to furniture.*

i) Why is she not crawling?

ii) Is her motor development within the normal range?

5. i)

   ii) Yes ❑ No ❑

6. *A paediatrician is asked to see Charlie, aged 18 months, because his mother is concerned that he is not walking. Her other children walked before they were a year old. Assessment of his fine motor skills and vision shows that he scribbles with a pencil. He is able to build a tower of three bricks. He has a vocabulary of around 20 words and clearly understands simple commands. He is able to feed himself with a spoon and tries to undress himself.*

i) Apart from his gross motor skills, is his development within normal limits?

ii) List the three most likely reasons why he is not walking:

6. i) Yes ❑ No ❑
   ii)

7. *Lucie is noted to perform the following tasks:*

Gross motor – she can kick a ball

Fine motor skills/vision – she can build a bridge with bricks when shown and is able to draw a circle

Language/hearing – she speaks well in sentences

Social and self-help skills/behaviour – she points to several different parts of her body as specified. She likes pretending to be a nurse. She eats with a knife and fork.

Select the minimum age at which she is likely to be able to perform all these tasks:

A 1 year

B 1$\frac{1}{2}$ years

C 2 years

D 3 years

E 4$\frac{1}{2}$ years

7. A B C D E

8. *A health visitor is concerned about a 19-month-old girl. She is still only babbling and says no distinct words. She is able to walk, scribbles with crayons and attempts to feed herself with a spoon.*

What is the first test to request?

8.

9. *Charlotte, aged four months, is referred because of constant crying and poor feeding. She is fed on milk alone. Her mother tearfully complains that she is finding it very difficult to cope. She also has a 20-month-old boy who has recently been referred to the speech and language therapist because of language delay. She used to work as a solicitor and her partner is a company director who often travels abroad. Charlotte's clinical and developmental examination and growth are normal.*

What family factor is the likeliest cause of this infant's problems?

9.

10.

Select the most appropriate description of the audiograms below from each of the following:

A   The hearing loss of the right ear is: sensorineural/conductive/mixed

B   The bilateral hearing loss is: sensorineural/conductive/mixed

A

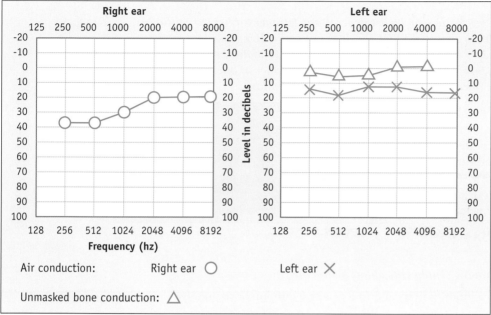

Fig. 3.1

B

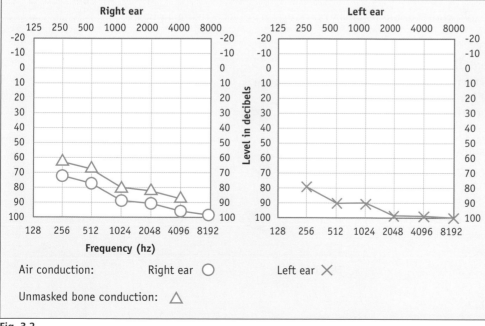

Fig. 3.2

11. *Which of the following statements about hearing are true or false:*

A A normal newborn infant startles to loud noises

B A newborn infant of a mother with sensorineural hearing loss should be booked for a distraction hearing test at 7–9 months

C A four-month-old infant who babbles has normal hearing

D An eight-month-old infant should turn to sounds out of his line of vision

E Secretory otitis media (glue ear) is the commonest reason for failing the eight-month distraction test

11.

A True ❏   False ❏

B True ❏   False ❏

C True ❏   False ❏

D True ❏   False ❏

E True ❏   False ❏

12. *Jenny, aged eight weeks, is seen by her general practitioner for her surveillance review. Her mother is concerned that she does not smile. Her gross motor development appears to be normal and she startles to loud noises. However she will not follow a face nor a colourful ball. The appearance of one of her eyes is shown in Fig. 3.3; the appearance of the other eye is similar.*

A What abnormality is shown?

B How might this condition have been detected earlier?

C What would be your initial management of this infant?

12. A

B

C

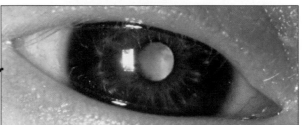

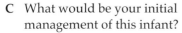

Fig. 3.3

13. *Which of the following statements about vision are true or false:*

A A normal newborn infant will fix and follow a face moving horizontally

B An infant of six months with a squint should be referred for a specialist ophthalmological opinion

C Cataracts are the commonest cause of squints

D A non-paralytic convergent squint causes double vision

E A normal one-year-old child should be able to pick up tiny objects using a pincer grip

13.

A True ❏   False ❏

B True ❏   False ❏

C True ❏   False ❏

D True ❏   False ❏

E True ❏   False ❏

14. *Katrina, aged 21 months, is asked to look at the observer's nose directly in front of her (A). The left eye is covered (B) and then uncovered (C).*

i) Is this a paralytic squint?

ii) What is the diagnosis?

14. i)

ii)

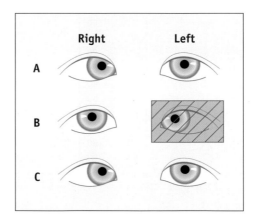

Fig. 3.4

15. *What is amblyopia?*

15.

1. Developmental milestones

		Median age			
		6 weeks	3 months	6 months	12 months
A	Sits unsupported			✓	
B	Reaches for objects		✓		
C	Smiles responsively	✓			
D	Says one or two single words with meaning				✓
E	Walks unsupported				✓

2.
A   *False.* An infant would only roll over at about four months.
B   *True.*
C   *True.*
D   *True.* This is the grasp reflex.
E   *False.* This occurs from six months.

3.
i)   Hand preference. This is abnormal before one year of age.
ii) Cerebral palsy with right hemiplegia. Detailed neurological examination is required to confirm this.

4.
A   *False.* The median age is 14 months.
B   *True.* The median age is 10 months.
C   *True.*
D   *False.* The child will need to be $1^1/_2$ years old to do this.
E   *False.* The median age is 18 months.

5.
i)   She is bottom shuffling, a locomotor variant.
ii) Yes.

6.
i)   Yes.
ii) Variant of normal
     Cerebral palsy
     Neuromuscular disorder e.g. Duchenne muscular dystrophy

7.   D – 3 years

8.   A hearing test.

9.   Maternal depression. This is likely to have a profound effect on her baby's development as infants are totally dependent on their carer.

10.
A – conductive hearing loss. The hearing loss on the right is mild (30–50 dBHL) and conductive as high frequency hearing is relatively preserved and bone conduction is normal.
B – sensorineural hearing loss. The hearing loss is severe (70–90 dBHL) to profound (> 90 dBHL) and sensorineural as there is no significant air–bone gap.

11.
A   *True.*
B   *False.* The infant should be promptly referred for audiological assessment soon after birth, otherwise the opportunity for early amplification and assistance will be lost. The distraction test cannot be used at this age.
C   *False.* Infants with severe hearing loss may still babble.
D   *True.* This is the basis of the distraction hearing test performed at this age.
E   *True.* Sensorineural hearing loss is much less common.

12.
A   Cataract.
B   Checking for red reflex during the newborn examination.
C   Urgent specialist ophthalmological referral. Delay in treatment is likely to lead to permanent visual loss.

13. **A** *True.*
    B *True.*
    C *False.* Although a cataract may cause a squint, refractive errors are the commonest cause.
    D *False.* Double vision does not occur with non-paralytic squints because of suppression of the image from the squinting eye.
    E *True.*

14. i) No. The right eye moves to fixate the object when the left eye is covered.
    ii) Right convergent squint.

15. Amblyopia is the failure of development of visual acuity in an eye that has been prevented from seeing (e.g. by a squint or cataract) early in life.

4 Care of the sick child

1. *Which of the following statements are true or false:*

A   The majority of paediatric medical admissions are school-aged children.

B   The majority of surgical admissions are infants.

C   Day-care surgery is best avoided in young children.

D   Respiratory disorders are the commonest reason for paediatric medical admission to hospital.

E   A child admitted under a general surgeon should also have a named consultant paediatrician responsible for their care.

2. *Complete the table with ticks matching the most appropriate pain management strategy with each of the following case histories. More than one strategy may apply.*

Pain managing strategies:

A   Distraction

B   Topical anaesthetic

C   Regular non-steroidal anti-inflammatory drug (NSAID) e.g. ibuprofen

D   Morphine via a nurse-controlled pump

E   Patient-controlled analgesia (PCA) with morphine

F   Regular oral long-acting morphine with rapid action oromorph for breakthrough pain

	Pain strategy					
	A	B	C	D	E	F
1 A three-year-old boy attending outpatients who requires a blood test						
2 A four-year-old boy who has had a thoracotomy						
3 A 13-year-old boy with a sickle cell crisis complaining of severe pain in his left leg						
4 A 10-year-old boy with severe pain from metastatic Ewing's sarcoma which is unresponsive to therapy						

3. *Which of the following statements about drug prescribing are true or false:*

A   In a vomiting child all medication must be given intravenously

B   In infants, regular intramuscular injections are preferable to the intravenous route as siting a cannula is difficult

C   A six-year old child should be prescribed medicines in tablet form to ease their administration

D   In neonates the half-life of many drugs is increased because of their low glomerular filtration rate (GFR) and immature liver enzymes

E   With an intravenous aminoglycoside, e.g. gentamicin, trough plasma concentration measurements should be performed even in neonates and young children

1. **A** *False.* The majority of paediatric medical admissions are infants and pre-school children.
   B *False.* The majority of paediatric surgical admissions are school aged.
   C *False.* Most surgery in young children is done as day cases to avoid the emotional upset of an overnight stay. It also reduces the cost.
   D *True.*
   E *True.* In the UK, this is required under the Patients' Charter.

2.

		A	B	C	D	E	F
1	A three-year-old boy attending outpatients who requires a blood test	✓	✓				
2	A four-year-old boy who has had a thoracotomy				✓		
3	A 13-year-old boy with a sickle cell crisis complaining of severe pain in his left leg			✓		✓	
4	A 10-year-old boy with severe pain from metastatic Ewing's sarcoma which is unresponsive to therapy			✓			✓

3. **A** *False.* Medication can also be given rectally.
   B *False.* Intramuscular injections should be avoided if at all possible as they are painful and there is little muscle bulk for injection.
   C *False.* Young children find tablets difficult to take.
   D *True.*
   E *True.* This is especially important in neonates as they have a low GFR. The trough level is to ensure adequate gentamicin clearance prior to the next dose.

5 Paediatric emergencies

1. *Ryan, aged ten months, is rushed to the Accident and Emergency department after being found submerged in the bath. The paramedical team are giving him cardiopulmonary resuscitation.*

   i) Which of the following statements are true or false:

   A 100% oxygen should be given

   B In managing the airway, his head should be in the neutral position

   C The ratio of chest compressions to breaths is 5:1

   D A prolonged capillary refill time is a feature of shock

   E Cardiac compressions can be stopped when his brachial pulse first becomes palpable

   Ryan is intubated and given artificial ventilation with oxygen. Cardiac compressions are continued.

   ii) Which of the following diagrams shows a correct way of giving chest compressions in this infant and why?

   A   **B**   **C**

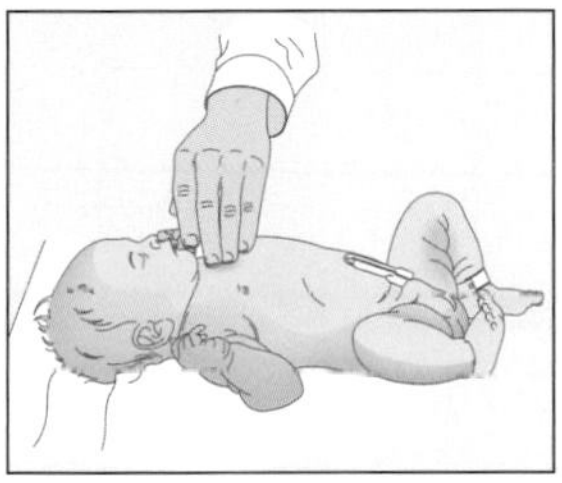

   Fig. 5.1   Fig. 5.2   Fig. 5.3

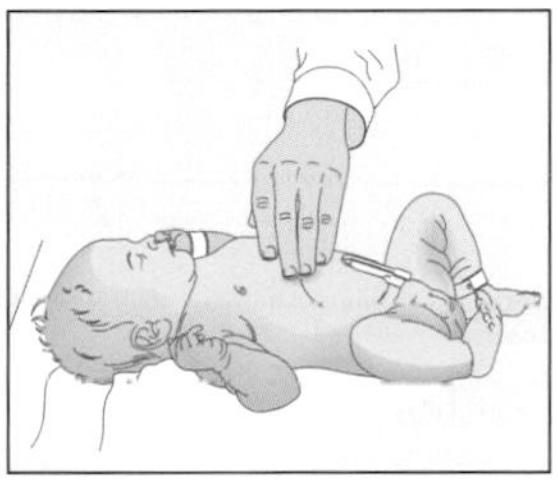

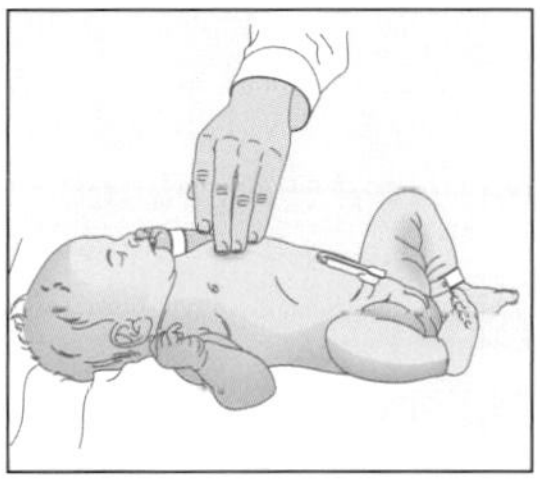

   iii) Three brief attempts at peripheral intravenous cannulation are unsuccessful. How would you gain circulatory access?

   iv) His ECG monitor shows asystole. Which drug is indicated?

   v) After 30 min cardiopulmonary resuscitation, Ryan remains asystolic. His rectal temperature is 29°C. Is it appropriate to withdraw life support?

2. *Complete the table below giving two examples of the causes of shock in each category.*

Hypovolaemia	
Maldistribution of fluid	

Answer column

1. i)

   A True ☐ False ☐

   B True ☐ False ☐

   C True ☐ False ☐

   D True ☐ False ☐

   E True ☐ False ☐

   ii) **A B C**

   iii)

   iv)

   v) Yes ☐ No ☐

3. *Mohammed, aged eight months, has been vomiting and off his feeds for two days. Initially he had episodes of crying uncontrollably, drawing his legs up into his abdomen as if in pain, and appeared fractious. His mother gave him some oral rehydration solution but his vomiting continued and he has become lethargic. On admission to hospital he is in shock.*

i) Which intravenous fluid would you give immediately?

ii) His weight is 8 kg. What volume of fluid would you give initially? Select the most appropriate from the list below.

A 40 ml

B 160 ml

C 320 ml

D 680 ml

E 800 ml

iii) What is his total fluid requirement for the initial 24 hours? Assume he is 10% dehydrated. The maintenance intravenous fluid requirement for a child of this age is 100 ml/kg/24 h. His plasma sodium is 138 mmol/l. His continuing fluid loss from vomiting is small and can be ignored.

A 160 ml

B 320 ml

C 800 ml

D 880 ml

E 1600 ml

His stool was noted to be mixed with blood.

iv) What is the likely diagnosis?

4. *Which of the following statements about status epilepticus are true or false:*

A It is defined as a convulsion which continues for at least one hour

B The immediate management is to give diazepam rectally or intravenously

C A blood glucose should be measured urgently

D An urgent anti-convulsant level is required

E Artificial ventilation is required if the convulsion fails to respond to anti-convulsant drugs

5. *Most febrile illnesses are mild viral infections. In a febrile child, which of the following are suggestive of a more serious illness:*

A Age less than two months old

B A low neutrophil count

C A low acute phase reactant, e.g. C-reactive protein

D A history of recurrent upper respiratory tract infections

E A history of long-term oral steroid treatment

3. i)

   ii) A B C D E
   iii) A B C D E
   iv)

4.
A True ❑ False ❑
B True ❑ False ❑
C True ❑ False ❑
D True ❑ False ❑
E True ❑ False ❑

5.
A True ❑ False ❑
B True ❑ False ❑
C True ❑ False ❑
D True ❑ False ❑
E True ❑ False ❑

6. *Samantha, aged four years, develops a fever and lethargy. She is given paracetamol but goes to bed complaining that she is aching all over and has a headache. Some hours later she is unrousable and is rushed to hospital. Her breathing is noted to be shallow, she is unresponsive to commands but withdraws her leg in response to a painful stimulus. No rash is visible. Her temperature is 38.2°C, her pulse 120/min and blood pressure 100/50. Her capillary refill time is 2 sec.*

i) List two likely diagnoses.

ii) Would you quickly do a lumbar puncture? Justify your decision.

iii) List two important therapeutic interventions.

7. *Which of the following statements about the death of a child are true or false:*

A Sudden Infant Death Syndrome (SIDS) is defined as the unexpected death of an infant.

B Sudden Infant Death Syndrome (SIDS) predominantly affects infants of 1–6 months.

C Sleeping supine reduces the risk of Sudden Infant Death Syndrome (SIDS).

D Following a fatal accident, parents should be discouraged from seeing their child.

E Grief may be manifest by behavioural problems in the siblings of a child who has died.

6. i)

ii)

iii)

7.

A True ❏ False ❏

B True ❏ False ❏

C True ❏ False ❏

D True ❏ False ❏

E True ❏ False ❏

1. i) **A** *True.*
    B *True.* Over-extension of the neck in infants will obstruct the airway.
    C *True.*
    D *True.* The capillary refill time is determined by pressing on the pulp of a digit for 5 sec, causing it to blanche, and timing the return of the circulation. Normal is considered to be ≤ 2 sec. The sign is affected by skin temperature and should not be considered in isolation.
    E *False.* Cardiac compressions must be continued until the pulse rate is > 60/min.
    ii) **B.** In an infant, the heart is lower in relation to the external landmarks than in older children or adults and the area of compression over the sternum should be one fingerbreadth below an imaginary line between the nipples.
    iii) Intraosseous needle (Fig. 5.4)
    iv) Epinephrine (adrenaline). This is given intravenously, via an intraosseous infusion or down the endotracheal tube.
    v) No. He needs to be warmed until his core temperature is at least 32°C. Below this temperature, failure to respond to resuscitation may be due to the hypothermia. Furthermore, the hypothermia may also protect the brain and other organs from hypoxic damage.

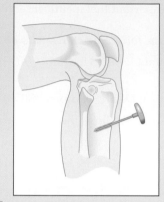

Fig. 5.4

2. Examples of the causes of shock are:

Hypovolaemia	Dehydration – gastroenteritis, diabetic ketoacidosis
	Blood loss – trauma
	Plasma loss – burns, nephrotic syndrome
Maldistribution of fluid	Septicaemia
	Anaphylaxis
	Bowel obstruction

3. i) 0.9% saline or colloid
    ii) **B.** This is 20 ml/kg initially, repeated as necessary
    iii) **E.** This is calculated by adding:
    Deficit: 10% of 8 kg = 800 ml
    Maintenance: 100 ml/kg/24 h = 800 ml
    Continuing losses: 0 ml
    Total: 1600 ml
    iv) Intussusception

4. **A** *False.* Status epilepticus is defined as a continuous seizure or multiple seizures with no waking between them, lasting more than 30 min.
    B *False.* The immediate management is of **A**irway, **B**reathing and **C**irculation.
    C *True.*
    D *False.* This will not influence the immediate management, but may help in monitoring drug dosage for some anti-convulsants and in assessing compliance.
    E *True.*

5. A *True.* Infants under two months' months who become febrile have a high incidence of bacterial infection.
   B *True.*
   C *False.* A high CRP suggests a bacterial infection. However, the CRP may be normal early in a bacterial infection.
   D *False.* These are common and rarely indicate an underlying immunodeficiency.
   E *True.* This will impair the immune response.

6. i) Conditions to be considered in a febrile, unconscious child are:
       Septicaemia/bacterial meningitis
       Viral meningitis/encephalitis
       Post-ictal
       Less likely diagnoses in a febrile child are:
       Metabolic disorder, e.g. diabetic ketoacidosis, hypoglycaemia, Reye's syndrome and inborn errors of metabolism
       Drug/poison ingestion
       Intracranial haemorrhage
   ii) No. Her condition is too unstable and she may have raised intracranial pressure.
   iii) Intubate and give artificial ventilation to support her breathing and protect her airway
       Intravenous antibiotic therapy
       Intravenous aciclovir in case she has herpes simplex encephalitis

7. A *False.* SIDS is defined as a sudden and unexpected death for which no adequate cause is found on a thorough autopsy.
   B *True.* The risk is highest at 2–4 months of age.
   C *True.* Sleeping prone, overheating and exposure to smoke antenatally or postnatally place infants at increased risk.
   D *False.* Most (but not all) parents find that seeing and holding their child helps with their grieving.
   E *True.*

6 Environment

1. *Which of the following statements about accidents are true or false:*

A They are the commonest cause of death in children aged 1 to 14 years in the UK

B In the UK they are responsible for more deaths per year than 10 years ago

C Falls are the commonest cause of fatal accidents in children

D They are commoner in lower socio-economic groups

E Small children held securely by an adult in the back of a car do not require a seat belt

2. *Tom, aged three years, fell from a first-floor balcony on to a concrete path. He immediately cried out in pain, but appeared to be all right. He was brought to the Accident and Emergency department by his parents after vomiting several times. On examination he is found to be fully conscious but has a large bruise over the left parietal region.*

i) Select the most serious clinical sign:

    A Nasal discharge since his fall

    B Further enlargement of the parietal bruise

    C A fractured nose

    D Laceration above the eye requiring suturing

    E A unilateral black eye

There are no focal neurological signs nor any other injuries. This is the lateral skull X-ray (Fig. 6.1).

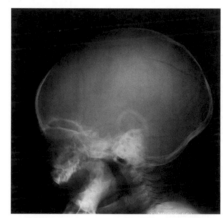

Fig. 6.1

ii) What does it show?

Eight hours after admission, the nurses note a change in his level of consciousness. He is now responsive only to painful stimuli; his left pupil is dilated although still responsive to light. His airway, breathing and circulation are satisfactory. A CT scan is performed (Fig. 6.2).

iii) List two abnormalities.

iv) Which of the following is the most appropriate immediate management:

    A Clotting studies

    B Skeletal survey

    C Ophthalmology opinion

    D Neurosurgical referral

    E EEG

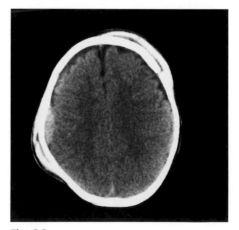

Fig. 6.2

1.

A True ❑ False ❑

B True ❑ False ❑

C True ❑ False ❑

D True ❑ False ❑

E True ❑ False ❑

2. i) A B C D E

  ii)

  iii)

  iv) A B C D E

3. *Louise, aged four years, was hit by a car in the local supermarket car park. She is brought to the Accident and Emergency department by the paramedical team. An initial assessment shows:*

Airway   – neck collar in place, talking to mother

Breathing   – receiving oxygen via a rebreathing circuit, oxygen saturation 99%
            – air entry satisfactory and equal bilaterally, respiratory rate 30/min

Circulation – pulse 160/min, blood pressure 90/50, capillary refill time 3 sec

Disability – Alert but frightened and agitated, moving all four limbs.

She has abrasions to her left flank and pain in her left shoulder.

i)   What intervention is required immediately?

ii) What is required before her cervical spine support can safely be removed?

Chest and abdominal X-rays show fractures of the 9th and 10th ribs on the left side.

iii) What is the most likely cause of this girl's hypovolaemic shock?

iv) How would you confirm your diagnosis?

4. *Ronaldo, aged 2½ years, pulled a chip pan off the cooker and has been extensively burnt. He is rushed to the nearest Accident and Emergency department. His airway, breathing and circulation are satisfactory. His burns are shown on the chart below. Most of the burnt area is now blistering and mottled in colour, with a few white areas. Intravenous analgesia is given.*

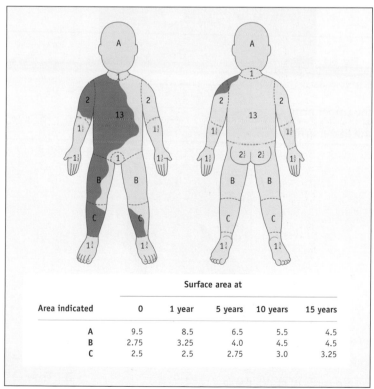

Area indicated	Surface area at				
	0	1 year	5 years	10 years	15 years
A	9.5	8.5	6.5	5.5	4.5
B	2.75	3.25	4.0	4.5	4.5
C	2.5	2.5	2.75	3.0	3.25

Fig. 6.3

3. i)

   ii)

   iii)

   iv)

4. i)   A B C D E
   ii) A B C D E
   iii)

   iv) Yes ❏   No ❏

i) Estimate the area of the burn, selecting your answer from the list below:

  A 10%

  B 20%

  C 40%

  D 60%

  E 80%

ii) What immediate management does he require?

  Select the most important item from the list below:

  A Intravenous 0.9% saline or colloid

  B Place in cold water

  C Cover the burns with sterile dressings

  D Intubation and artificial ventilation

  E Intravenous antibiotics

iii) Why is specialist care required?

iv) Is this likely to be an example of child abuse?

5. *This child is said to have pulled a kettle of boiling water over her legs. Are the injuries compatible with this history?*

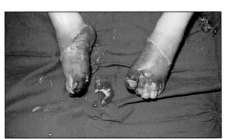

Fig. 6.4

5. Yes ❑ No ❑

6. *Fig. 6.5*

i) What is the cause of the lesion on the upper arm?

ii) What is the cause of the lesion on the lower arm?

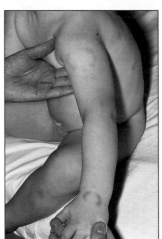

Fig. 6.5

6. i)

   ii)

7. *Which of these statements about poisoning are true or false:*

A It is the commonest cause of fatal accident in children

B Most ingestions of tablets in toddlers are cases of child abuse

C Emesis with ipecac is contraindicated following ingestion of corrosives and petroleum distillates

D Activated charcoal is contraindicated in young children

E The incidence of salicylate ingestion is less than it was 15 years ago

7.

A True ❑ False ❑

B True ❑ False ❑

C True ❑ False ❑

D True ❑ False ❑

E True ❑ False ❑

8. *Complete the table below indicating whether the substance is of high or low potential toxicity if ingested:*

Substance	High toxicity	Low toxicity
Petroleum product, e.g. white spirit		
Oral contraceptive pill		
Washing powder		
Laburnum		
Penicillin		

9. *Which of the following statements about the complications of poisoning in children are true or false:*

A Cardiac dysrrhythmias are a recognised complication of tricyclic anti-depressant ingestion

B Salicylate poisoning may result in a metabolic alkalosis

C Acetylcysteine reduces the risk of liver failure in paracetamol ingestion

D Alcohol ingestion is associated with hyperglycaemia

E An ingested screw or nail should immediately be surgically removed

9.

A True ❑   False ❑
B True ❑   False ❑
C True ❑   False ❑
D True ❑   False ❑
E True ❑   False ❑

10. *Solomon, aged 2½ years, has been found eating some of his pregnant mother's iron tablets; up to 10 tablets are missing. Their general practitioner advised that he should be taken to hospital directly. On examination he is found to be talkative, with no obvious abnormalities.*

i) Select the investigation you would perform first:

   A Abdominal X-ray

   B Full blood count

   C Clotting studies

   D Serum iron

   E Liver function tests

ii) Your investigation suggests a significant ingestion. Which of the following would you initiate? More than one may be correct.

   A Intravenous acetylcysteine

   B Intravenous naloxone

   C Intravenous desferrioxamine

   D Forced alkaline diuresis

   E Intubate and hyperventilate

10. i) A B C D E
ii) A True ❑ False ❑
    B True ❑ False ❑
    C True ❑ False ❑
    D True ❑ False ❑
    E True ❑ False ❑

11. This six-year-old boy caught a 5p coin in his mouth.

i) Describe the abnormality seen in the chest X-ray.

ii) How would you manage this problem?

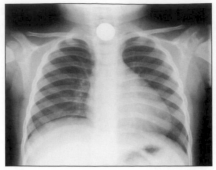

Fig. 6.6

12. *Chelsea, aged two years, was playing ball at home with her mother's partner when she tumbled down a flight of seven stairs. Her mother brought her directly to the Accident and Emergency department where she is noted to have a swollen thigh and refuses to walk. She has no other injuries. Her growth and development are normal for age. X-ray reveals oblique midshaft fracture of her left femur. Her leg is splinted and an X-ray taken (Fig. 6.7).*

i) Is the type of fracture consistent with the history given?

Six months later Chelsea is brought to the Accident and Emergency department by her mother. She said that Chelsea had slipped in the bath while briefly left alone. On examination there is swelling and bruising over Chelsea's anterior right chest wall. She has some older bruises on her right thigh.

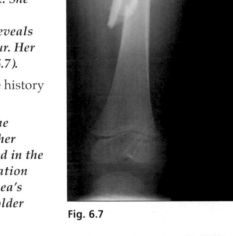

Fig. 6.7

ii) A chest X-ray is taken (Fig. 6.8). What abnormality does it show?

iii) Select the most likely explanation for Chelsea's injuries:

  A Osteogenesis imperfecta

  B Bone tumour

  C Non-accidental injury

  D Haemophilia B

  E Vitamin D deficiency

iv) Select the most appropriate management:

  A Genetic counselling

  B Intravenous antibiotics

  C Parental reassurance

  D Child protection case conference

  E None of the above

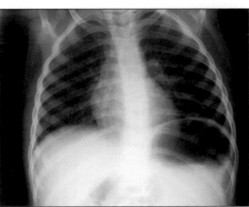

Fig. 6.8

11. i)

    ii)

12. i)   Yes ❑   No ❑
    ii)

    iii)   **A B C D E**
    iv)   **A B C D E**

13. *Pauline, who is six years old, alleges to her teacher that her stepfather hurt her with his 'willy'. She is seen by the consultant paediatrician who does not find any abnormalities on examination.*

i) Are the examination findings compatible with the diagnosis of sexual abuse?

ii) Which of the following findings would be suggestive of sexual abuse?

   A Gonococcal infection

   B Vulval soreness

   C Sexualised behaviour

   D Precocious breast development

   E Bruising to the thighs

i) Yes ❏   No ❏

ii)

A True ❏   False ❏

B True ❏   False ❏

C True ❏   False ❏

D True ❏   False ❏

E True ❏   False ❏

1. **A** *True.*
   B *False.* There has been a marked reduction.
   C *False.* Road traffic accidents are the commonest, followed by fires, drowning and suffocation.
   D *True.*
   E *False.* All children in cars must be secured in a car-seat or with a seatbelt.

2. i) **A.** This may be CSF leakage from a basal skull fracture.
   ii) Left parietal fracture.

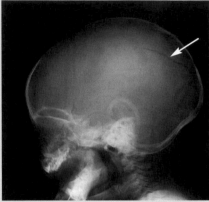

Fig. 6.9

iii)

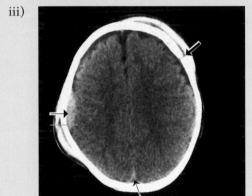

Skull fracture ↑
Subdural haematoma ↑ and blood in falx ↑.

Fig. 6.10

   iv) **D.**

3. i) Intravenous access and volume to treat her shock. She should also be given analgesia.
   ii) Normal neurological examination and normal cervical spine X-rays.
   iii) Splenic injury.
   iv) Immediate abdominal ultrasound/CT scan or diagnostic peritoneal lavage.

4. i) **B.**
   ii) **A.**
      Placing in cold water is useful for pain relief for small burns.
      Covering the burns is not urgent.
      Intubation and ventilation is not required as the airway and breathing are satisfactory.
      Intravenous antibiotics are not needed urgently.
   iii) The burn is greater than 10% and there are areas of full thickness burns which will probably require skin graft.
   iv) No. The injuries are consistent with the history and he was brought immediately to Accident and Emergency. However one would need further information about how and why the accident actually happened and about the child's supervision. Further information is also required about past accidents within the family. This information may be obtained from the health visitor or GP.

5. No. These scalds are caused by placing the child in very hot water.

6. i) A bite mark from an adult.
    ii) A bite mark from a child.

7. **A** *False.* Poisoning is rarely fatal in children.
    B *False.* Most poisoning in toddlers is accidental, by inquisitive toddlers unaware of the potential danger.
    C *True.*
    D *False.*
    E *True.* This is because aspirin is rarely prescribed for children (because of the association with Reye syndrome) and the use of childproof containers for medications.

8. | Substance | High toxicity | Low toxicity |
    |---|---|---|
    | Petroleum product, e.g. white spirit | ✓ | |
    | Oral contraceptive pill | | ✓ |
    | Washing powder | | ✓ |
    | Laburnum | ✓ | |
    | Penicillin | | ✓ |

9. **A** *True.*
    B *False.* It results in a metabolic acidosis.
    C *True.*
    D *False.* Alcohol ingestion is association with hypoglycaemia.
    E *False.* Most screws or nails will be passed uneventfully. Surgical or endoscopic removal may be required if they do not pass beyond the pylorus.

10. i) A. This identifies if there is a significant number of tablets in his stomach. The serum iron will not be helpful at this early stage.
     ii) **A** *False.* This is the antidote for paracetamol poisoning.
          B *False.* This is the antidote for opiate poisoning.
          C *True.*
          D *False.* This may be performed for salicylate poisoning.
          E *False.*

11.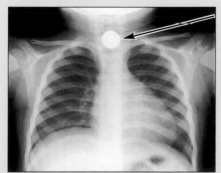

     i) There is a 5p coin stuck in the upper oesophagus. It lies just above the cricopharyngeus muscle.
     ii) Remove it endoscopically.

Fig. 6.11

12. i) Yes.
    ii) Rib fractures (5th, 6th and 7th ribs on the right).
    iii) **C.**
    iv) **D.**

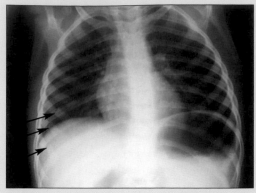

Fig. 6.12

13. i) Yes. Significant abnormal physical findings are observed in less than a third of substantiated cases.
    ii) **A** *True.*
        B *False.* This is common in young girls.
        C *True.*
        D *False.*
        E *True.*

7 Genetics

1. *Fig. 7.1*

i) The midwife suspects that this newborn infant may have Down's syndrome. List three craniofacial features you would look for to support this diagnosis.

ii) Children with Down's syndrome are at increased risk of which of the following:

  A Hypothyroidism

  B Secretory otitis media

  C Coeliac disease

  D Talipes

  E Cataracts

iii) A murmur is heard at 10 days of age. Select the most likely cardiac lesion from the list below:

  A Atrio-ventricular septal defect

  B Patent ductus arteriosus

  C Coarctation of the aorta

  D Pulmonary stenosis

  E Tetralogy of Fallot

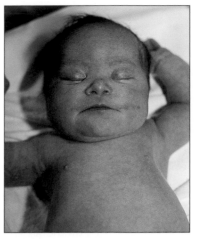

Fig. 7.1

2. *A couple attend genetic counselling after their first child is born with Down's syndrome.*

i) Select the most likely genetic mechanism to have been responsible:

  A Non-disjunction

  B Translocation

  C Mosaicism

  D Point mutation

  E Triplet repeat expansion

Their baby's chromosomes are examined. Three copies of chromosome 21 are seen, one of which is attached to chromosome 14.

ii) How would you describe this abnormality?

  A Non-disjunction

  B Balanced translocation

  C Unbalanced translocation

  D Mosaicism

  E Triplet repeat expansion

iii) What implications does this have for future pregnancies?

---

1. i)

ii)

  A True ☐   False ☐

  B True ☐   False ☐

  C True ☐   False ☐

  D True ☐   False ☐

  E True ☐   False ☐

iii)

2. i)   A B C D E

  ii)   A B C D E

  iii)

3. *Place a tick in the table of clinical features of Down's, Kleinfelter's and Fragile X syndromes as appropriate. More than one or none may apply.*

Clinical feature	Down's syndrome	Kleinfelter's	Fragile X
A Duodenal atresia			
B Abnormal size testes (in adolescence)			
C Infertility			
D Short stature			
E Hearing impairment from secretory otitis media			

4. *Which of the following statements about autosomal dominant inheritance are true or false:*

A The chance of inheriting an abnormal gene from an affected parent is 1 in 4 (25%)

B The absence of a family history excludes this form of inheritance

C An individual with the gene defect may be asymptomatic

D The abnormal gene is never carried on the sex chromosomes

E The risk diminishes with successive pregnancies

4.

A True ❑ False ❑

B True ❑ False ❑

C True ❑ False ❑

D True ❑ False ❑

E True ❑ False ❑

5. *Gemma and Mark, who are both well, are planning to start a family. Gemma's older brother has cystic fibrosis but her two sisters are unaffected. Mark is an only child. There is no history of cystic fibrosis in his family.*

i) Draw their pedigree.

5.

ii) What is Gemma's risk of being a carrier?

iii) What is the risk of Gemma and Mark having a child with cystic fibrosis (assume the carrier rate is 1 in 25)?

ii)

iii)

6. *Which of the following statements about autosomal recessive inheritance are true or false:*

A Males and females are equally likely to be affected

B The abnormal gene is most likely to code for a structural protein

C Both parents must be carriers to have an affected child

D Is excluded by an absent family history

E Consanguinity increases the risk of the disorder

6.

A True ❑ False ❑

B True ❑ False ❑

C True ❑ False ❑

D True ❑ False ❑

E True ❑ False ❑

7. *Which of the following statements about X-linked recessive inheritance are true or false:*

A It never results in father to son transmission

B The abnormal genetic material is always carried on the X chromosome

C Daughters of affected males are always carriers

D It is less common than X-linked dominant inheritance

E Can result in both sexes showing clinical abnormalities

7.
A True ❑ False ❑
B True ❑ False ❑
C True ❑ False ❑
D True ❑ False ❑
E True ❑ False ❑

8. *Mark the type of inheritance against the following conditions.*

Conditions	Autosomal dominant	Autosomal recessive	X-linked recessive	Multifactorial
Pyloric stenosis				
Phenylketonuria				
Haemophilia A				
Achondroplasia				
Sickle cell disease				
Beta-thalassaemia major				
Neurofibromatosis				
Marfan's syndrome				
Developmental dysplasia of the hip				

9. *This child was floppy in the neonatal period and required tube feeding. Prader–Willi syndrome was suspected. The diagnosis was confirmed by genetic analysis when the child was found to have inherited both copies of the chromosome 15q11–13 region from his mother (Fig. 7.2).*

i) What is this form of genetic inheritance known as?

ii) What other genetic mechanism may cause this syndrome?

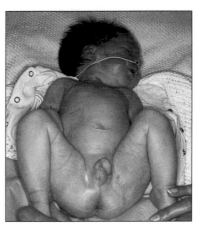

Fig. 7.2

9. i)

ii)

10. *A Jewish couple is referred for genetic counselling. Their three-year-old daughter died six months' earlier of Tay Sachs disease, an autosomal recessive deficiency of hexosaminidase A. The couple are first cousins. They are considering having another child.*

i) What is the risk of them having another affected baby?

ii) Which of the following are possible options for them to consider:

   A Testing both parents to confirm carrier status

   B Using artificial insemination by donor

   C Chorionic villus sampling and biochemical screening for levels of the enzyme

   D Detailed anomaly scan with the option of second trimester abortion

   E Have another child and hope for the best

iii) During genetic counselling, which option would you recommend to them?

10. i)

ii)

A True ❏   False ❏
B True ❏   False ❏
C True ❏   False ❏
D True ❏   False ❏
E True ❏   False ❏

iii) **A B C D E None**

11. i) What is the most likely pattern of inheritance shown here (Fig. 7.3)?

   ii) If the female marked with an arrow were a carrier, what would be the risk of her son being affected by the disorder?

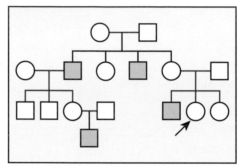

Fig. 7.3

11. i)

ii)

12. *Complete the table by selecting the common type of gene mutation responsible for the following disorders.*

Condition	Gene mutation	
	Trinucleotide repeat expansion	Gene deletion/ Point mutation
Fragile X		
Cystic fibrosis		
β-thalassaemia		
Huntington's disease		
Duchenne's muscular dystrophy		

13. *The grandfather of four-year-old Richard has recently been diagnosed as suffering from Huntington's disease. The boy's father is waiting for his test results. The family would like Richard to also be tested.*

Select the most appropriate management:

A Postpone testing until Richard is old enough to give informed consent

B Perform DNA analysis

C Perform chromosomal analysis

D Ultrasound scanning to visualise presymptomatic changes

E Fundoscopic examination by an ophthalmologist to visualise early signs

13. **A   B   C   D   E**

1. i)   Upslanting palpebral fissures
        Epicanthic folds
        Brushfield spots in iris
        Small mouth and relatively large tongue
        Small ears
        Flat occiput
    ii) **A** *True.*
        B *True.*
        C *False.*
        D *False.*
        E *True.*
    iii) **A**

2. i)   **A.** Non-disjunction. This is responsible for 94% of cases of Down's syndrome.
    ii) **C.** An unbalanced translocation.
    iii) An increased risk of recurrence as one of the parents is likely to have a balanced translocation
        whereby one of their copies of chromosome 21 is attached to chromosome 14.

3.

Clinical feature	Down's syndrome	Kleinfelter's	Fragile X
A Duodenal atresia	✓		
B Abnormal size testes		✓	✓
C Infertility		✓	
D Short stature	✓		
E Hearing impairment from secretory otitis media	✓		

4. **A** *False.* The risk is 1 in 2.
    B *False.* There is often, but not always, a family history. New mutations, gonadal mosaicism or
        non-paternity can be responsible for the absence of a family history.
    C *True.* There may be non-penetrance (where the abnormal gene is inherited but not expressed) or
        variable expression (clinical features may range from minimal to full).
    D *True.* Autosomal inheritance means that the abnormal gene is carried on one of a pair of autosomes
        (chromosomes 1–22)
    E *False.* The risk remains the same.

5. i)

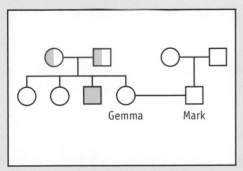

Fig. 7.4

    ii) 2 in 3. We know that Gemma does not have CF, therefore she has a 2/3 chance of being a carrier
        from simple Mendelian genetics.
    iii) 1:150. This is calculated as:

probability that Gemma is a carrier	×	probability that Mark is a carrier	×	probability of an affected child if they are both carriers
$= {}^2/_3$	×	$^1/_{25}$	×	$^1/_4$

$= {}^1/_{150}$

6.   **A**   *True.*
     B   *False.* This is true of autosomal dominant conditions.
     C   *True.* The risk of an affected child is 1 in 4 (25%).
     D   *False.*
     E   *True.* It increases the risk that the partners both carry the same defective gene inherited from a common ancestor.

7.   **A**   *True.* Fathers always transmit the Y chromosome to their sons.
     B   *True.*
     C   *True.* This is because they all receive the affected chromosome from their father.
     D   *False.* X-linked dominant conditions are very rare.
     E   *True.* Occasionally female carriers show signs of the disease.

8.

Conditions	Autosomal dominant	Autosomal recessive	X-linked recessive	Multi-factorial
Pyloric stenosis				✓
Phenylketonuria		✓		
Haemophilia A			✓	
Achondroplasia	✓			
Sickle cell disease		✓		
Beta-thalassaemia major		✓		
Neurofibromatosis	✓			
Marfan's syndrome	✓			
Development dysplasia of the hip				✓

9.   i)   Uniparental disomy.
    ii)   Deletion of the paternal chromosome 15q 11–13.

10.   i)   1 in 4.
    ii)   **A**   *False.* Both parents will be carriers as it is an autosomal recessive disorder.
         B   *True.*
         C   *True.*
         D   *False.* An affected fetus would not have any abnormalities detectable on ultrasound.
         E   *True.*
    iii)   None of them. Only the couple know which option is best for them. Genetic counselling should be non-directive.

11.   i)   X-linked recessive disorder.
    ii)   1 in 2. In an X-linked disorder, a female carrier will have one affected X chromosome. There is therefore a 1 in 2 chance of passing the affected X chromosome to any male offspring.

12.

Condition	Gene mutation	
	Trinucleotide repeat expansion	Gene deletion/Point mutation
Fragile X	✓	
Cystic fibrosis		✓
β-thalassaemia		✓
Huntington's disease	✓	
Duchenne's muscular dystrophy		✓

13. **A.** There is no treatment available to modify the course of the illness. Richard should therefore have the option of deciding whether or not to take a predictive test. This needs to be delayed until he is old enough to fully understand the implications. The disorder is diagnosed by DNA analysis. There are no physical abnormalities detectable in the presymptomatic phase.

8 Perinatal medicine

1. *Which of the following statements about perinatal care are true or false:*

   A Folic acid supplements should ideally be started as soon as a pregnancy test is positive.

   B If a mother smokes 20 cigarettes a day, she is likely to have a lighter infant than if she smokes five cigarettes a day.

   C A maternal serum screening test is available to tell if a fetus has Down's syndrome.

   D Abnormal nuchal translucency on an antenatal ultrasound scan is a feature of a neural tube defect.

   E Antenatal maternal glucocorticoid therapy reduces the incidence of respiratory distress syndrome in preterm infants.

1.

   A True ❏   False ❏

   B True ❏   False ❏

   C True ❏   False ❏

   D True ❏   False ❏

   E True ❏   False ❏

2. *This infant was born to a mother with insulin dependent diabetes.*

   i) What abnormality is shown?

   ii) List three other neonatal problems of which this infant is at increased risk.

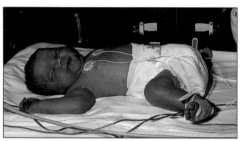

Fig. 8.1

2. i)

    ii)

3. *Callum is a two-day-old infant, birthweight 3.6 kg. He was born by vaginal delivery with Apgar scores of 7 at 1 minute and 10 at 5 minutes. On day 2, he is reported to be jittery, crying inconsolably and feeding poorly. He sneezes and yawns, and is thought to have some abnormal movements, possibly seizures.*

   Select the most likely explanation for Callum's problems

   A Congenital rubella syndrome

   B Fetal alcohol syndrome

   C Birth asphyxia

   D Kernicterus

   E Maternal opiate use

3. A   B   C   D   E

4. i) List three features of congenital rubella:

   ii) During which trimester does infection cause the most damage?

4. i)

    ii)

5. *A mother develops chicken pox (varicella) 24 hours after giving birth to a normal infant. From the list below select the most appropriate advice you would give.*

A Reassure and discharge home to avoid spread of infection

B Neonatal infection is unlikely due to transplacentally acquired antibodies

C There is a significant risk of serious neonatal infection

D Breast feeding is contraindicated

E The infant's varicella antibody status should be checked

6. *Which of the following statements about the normal cardiopulmonary changes following birth are true or false:*

A Pulmonary vascular resistance rises

B Blood flow across the foramen ovale increases in the first few hours of life compared to fetal life

C Flow of oxygenated blood across the patent ductus arteriosus causes it to close

D Increased left atrial filling occurs

E Fetal lung fluid secretion is reduced

7. *A newborn infant is noted at 1 minute of age to be centrally cyanosed and has occasional gasping respiration. His heart rate is 80 beats per minute and he grimaces and makes some weak flexion movements while being dried.*

i) What is his 1 minute Apgar score?

	Score		
	0	1	2
Appearance	Centrally white / blue	Blue peripherally Pink centrally	Pink
Pulse	0	<100	>100
Gasps (respiration)	Absent	Irregular	Regular
Activity (tone)	Limp	Decreased	Active
Reflex irritability (to pharangeal stimulation)	Nil	Grimace only	Strong coughs or cry

Maximum 10/10. Scored at 1 and 5 minutes unless still less than 9, in which case continue to score every 5 mins until ≥ 9.

ii) What, if anything, needs to be done for this baby?

iii) His condition deteriorates and his heart rate drops to 50 beats/min. What three immediate steps would you take?

Side column:

5. A B C D E

6.
A True ❑ False ❑
B True ❑ False ❑
C True ❑ False ❑
D True ❑ False ❑
E True ❑ False ❑

7.
i) Apgar score
ii)
iii)

8. *This infant required intubation and artificial ventilation shortly after birth for respiratory distress. At 20 minutes of age, his oxygen saturation remained poor. This is his chest X-ray.*

   What is the most likely diagnosis?

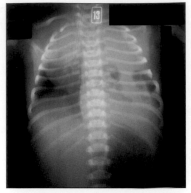

Fig. 8.2

8. i)

9. *These twins were born at 32 weeks' gestation.*

   List two of the problems of which the smaller twin is at increased risk in the immediate newborn period as a consequence of his growth restriction.

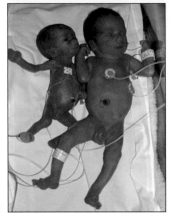

Fig. 8.3

9.

10. *Which of the following statements about newborn infants are true or false:*

   A The risk of developmental dysplasia of the hip (DDH, also known as congenital dislocation of the hip) is increased following a breech presentation

   B An absent red reflex is an indication for urgent ophthalmological referral

   C An undescended testis at routine neonatal examination is an indication for urgent surgical repair

   D A heart murmur heard on the first day of life is most likely to be due to congenital heart disease

   E Routine neonatal biochemical screening is performed on day 1 of life

10.

A True ❑ False ❑

B True ❑ False ❑

C True ❑ False ❑

D True ❑ False ❑

E True ❑ False ❑

11. *During a routine examination of a newborn boy, it is noted that he is not moving his left arm. He was born by vaginal delivery, birthweight 4.0 kg. He is feeding well and has no other neonatal problems.*

   What is the abnormality shown?

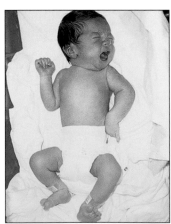

Fig. 8.4

11.

12. *Identify the lesions below. In each case, can spontaneous resolution be expected?*

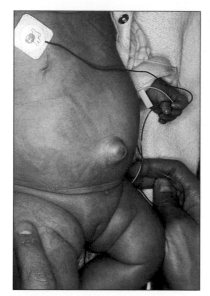

Fig. 8.5

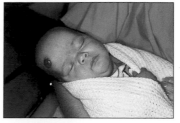

Fig. 8.6

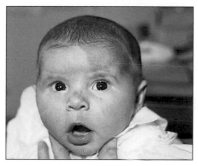

Fig. 8.7

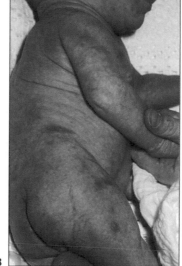

Fig. 8.8

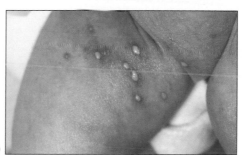

Fig. 8.9

12.

Resolve
spontaneously

Fig. 8.5

      Yes ❏   No ❏

Fig. 8.6

      Yes ❏   No ❏

Fig. 8.7

      Yes ❏   No ❏

Fig. 8.8

      Yes ❏   No ❏

Fig. 8.9

      Yes ❏   No ❏

13. *Why is it recommended that vitamin K should be given to all newborn infants?*

13.

1. A *False.* It is recommended that women should take folic acid before conception.
    B *True.*
    C *False.* The maternal serum screening test gives a risk of the fetus having Down's syndrome.
    D *False.* It is associated with Down's syndrome.
    E *True.*

2. i) Macrosomia.
    ii) Hypoglycaemia
        Respiratory distress syndrome
        Polycythaemia
        Congenital malformations
        Hypertrophic cardiomyopathy.

3. **E.** This history is characteristic of maternal opiate use.

    None of the commoner features of congenital rubella syndrome are present
    Infants with fetal alcohol syndrome are growth retarded and have characteristic facies
    Birth asphyxia could cause these neurological abnormalities but the sneezing, yawning and good
    Apgar scores at delivery are against this diagnosis
    Kernicterus is unlikely as severe jaundice is absent

4. i) **Common**
        Cataracts, congenital heart disease, deafness
        Growth retardation
        Uncommon
        Anaemia, thrombocytopenia
        Jaundice, hepatosplenomegaly
        Retinopathy, pneumonitis, encephalitis, bone lesions.
    ii) First trimester

5. **C.** If the mother develops chickenpox from five days before until 22 days after delivery, there will be insufficient time for protective antibodies to develop and be transferred to the infant. A quarter of such infants become infected with a significant mortality.

6. A *False.* As the lungs inflate there is a fall in pulmonary vascular resistance and therefore there is increased blood flow through the lungs.
    B *False.* Increased pressure in the left atrium causes the foramen ovale to close.
    C *True.*
    D *True.* This is because of increased pulmonary blood flow.
    E *True.*

7.

	Score		
	0	1	2
Appearance	Centrally white/blue	Blue peripherally Pink centrally	Pink
Pulse	0	<100	>100
Gasps (respiration)	Absent	Irregular	Regular
Activity (tone)	Limp	Decreased	Active
Reflex irritability (to pharangeal stimulation)	Nil	Grimace only	Strong coughs or cry

i) 4.
ii) He has not yet established regular respiration and is centrally cyanosed. He therefore needs immediate basic resuscitation to ensure a patent airway and mask ventilation should be started.

iii) Check that airway is clear and mask ventilation is optimal.
Call for help.
Start external cardiac massage.
Intubate and give artificial ventilation if unresponsive to above and expertise is available.

8. i) Left sided diaphragmatic hernia.

9. Birth asphyxia
Hypothermia
Hypoglycaemia
Polycythaemia.

10. **A** *True.*
B *True.*
C *False.* The majority descend spontaneously in the first year of life. It should be rechecked at several months of age.
D *False.* Most murmurs found at birth are innocent and will disappear within 72 h.
E *False.* It is performed at 5–9 days of age, after milk feeds have been established.

11. Left Erb's palsy.

12. Fig. 8.5   Umbilical hernia   Yes
Fig. 8.6   Strawberry naevus   Yes
Fig. 8.7   Port wine stain   No
Fig. 8.8   Erythema toxicum   Yes
Fig. 8.9   Septic spots   No

13. i) Newborn infants have low levels of vitamin K which puts them at risk of haemorrhagic disease of the newborn. Those at special risk are
Preterm infants
Exclusively breastfed infants
Infants with liver disease
Infants born to mothers on anti-convulsants

9 Neonatal medicine

1. *Which of the following statements about newborn infants are true or false:*
A An infant of birthweight 2.1 kg born at 37 weeks is classified as preterm
B An infant of birthweight 2.1 kg born at 37 weeks is classified as low birthweight
C Neonatal mortality is defined as the number of deaths in the first week of life per 1000 live births
D A stillbirth certificate should be issued for a 26-week gestation infant who is born with a heart rate of 120/min and irregular breathing but becomes asystolic at five minutes and dies in spite of resuscitation
E The commonest cause of death in the neonatal period is prematurity

2. *Which of the following statements about birth asphyxia are true or false:*
A It is defined as an Apgar score less than 3 at 1 minute of age
B A low Apgar score at 20 minutes of age is associated with an increased risk of long-term disability
C Irritability and hyperventilation are features of hypoxic ischaemic encephalopathy
D Recurrent seizures are a feature of mild hypoxic ischaemic encephalopathy
E Birth asphyxia is the commonest cause of cerebral palsy

3. *What abnormality is shown in each of these photographs?*

1.
A True ☐ False ☐
B True ☐ False ☐
C True ☐ False ☐
D True ☐ False ☐
E Truc ☐ False ☐

2.
A True ☐ False ☐
B True ☐ False ☐
C True ☐ False ☐
D True ☐ False ☐
E True ☐ False ☐

3. Fig. 9.1

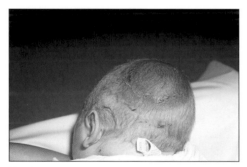

Fig. 9.1

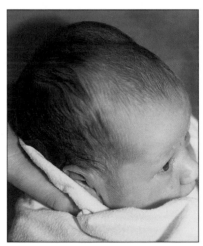

Fig. 9.2

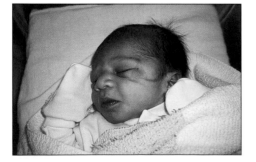

Fig. 9.3

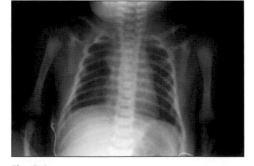

Fig. 9.4

Fig. 9.2

Fig. 9.3

Fig. 9.4

4. *Which of the following statements about preterm infants are true or false:*

A The gestational age can be estimated from the external appearance and neurological examination

B Surfactant promotes lung expansion by increasing surface tension

C Theophylline or caffeine are used to prevent episodes of apnoea and bradycardia

D They would be expected to be able to suck and swallow milk at 30–32 weeks' gestation

E Intraventricular haemorrhages most often occur in the first three days of life

5. *A preterm female infant, birthweight 725 g at 26 weeks' gestation, was given artificial ventilation immediately after birth, followed by surfactant via the tracheal tube. At four hours of age, when she was still requiring artificial ventilation and 80% oxygen, this chest X-ray was taken (Fig. 9.5).*

i) List two abnormal features on the chest X-ray.

ii) Select the most likely diagnosis based on the chest X-ray shown:

A Meconium aspiration

B Bronchopulmonary dysplasia

C Patent ductus arteriosus

D Respiratory distress syndrome

E Transient tachypnoea of the newborn

On the second day her condition suddenly deteriorated. A pneumothorax is suspected.

iii) List two clinical signs which would support this diagnosis.

iv) This is her chest X-ray. On which side is the pneumothorax?

A chest drain was inserted and her condition stabilised.

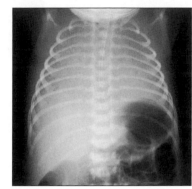

Fig. 9.5

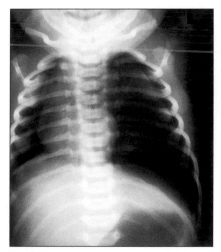

Fig. 9.6

4.

A True ❏ False ❏

B True ❏ False ❏

C True ❏ False ❏

D True ❏ False ❏

E True ❏ False ❏

5. i)

ii) A B C D E

iii)

iv)

Left ❏ Right ❏

Her cranial ultrasound scans at days 5 (Fig. 9.7) and 15 (Fig. 9.8) are shown.

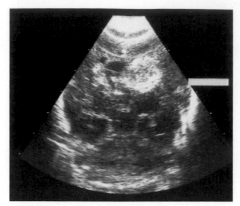

Fig. 9.7   Fig. 9.8

v) What do they show? Indicate the most appropriate answer in the table below.   v)

	Day 5	Day 15
A Normal		
B Intraventricular haemorrhage		
C Subdural haemorrhage		
D Ventricular dilatation		
E Periventricular leucomalacia		

6. *A male infant, birthweight 875 g at 28 weeks' gestation, required artificial ventilation for two weeks.*   6.

   At 10 weeks of age he is still needing additional oxygen via nasal cannulae. Fig. 9.9 shows his X-ray.

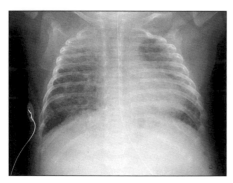

   Bronchopulmonary Dysplasia
   (chronic lung disease of
                   prematurity)

Fig. 9.9

   What is his lung condition called?

7. *Why might the oxygen tension in an arterial blood sample taken from a newborn infant's right arm differ from a sample taken from the left arm?*

8. *Robert is a full-term, male infant born at home. This was his mother's first pregnancy. At 16 hours of age it is noted that his skin and sclerae are yellow. He appears well and is taking some milk from the breast.*

i) Why would you investigate Robert's jaundice?

ii) What three investigations would you perform other than measuring the serum bilirubin?

His bilirubin was 150 μmol/l at 20 hours and he was given intensive phototherapy. Six hours later his bilirubin was 250 μmol/l (Fig. 9.10).

7.

8. i)

    ii)

    iii) **A B C D E**
    iv)

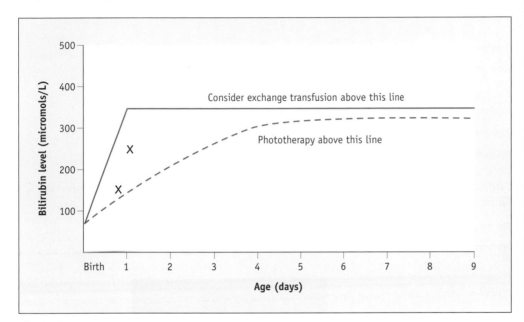

Fig. 9.10

iii) Select the most likely cause of his jaundice:

   A Physiological

   B Haemolysis, e.g. ABO incompatibility

   C Breast-milk jaundice

   D Biliary atresia

   E Congenital hypothyroidism

iv) What developmental function particularly needs to be checked following his severe jaundice?

9. *A midwife phones for advice about Grace, a three-day-old female Black-African term infant who has become jaundiced.*

i) List three further aspects of the history that you would want to know

The midwife checked the bilirubin level which was 200 (μmol/l (see bilirubin chart Fig. 9.10).

ii) Select the most likely cause of her jaundice:

    A Sickle cell disease

    B Rhesus incompatibility

    C Physiological

    D Hypothyroidism

    E Biliary atresia

iii) What is the most appropriate management?

    A Repeat bilirubin in 6 hours

    B Phototherapy

    C Exchange transfusion

    D Switch from breast to bottle feeding

    E Observation at home

10 *A full-term male infant, born by elective caesarean section, develops respiratory distress at two hours of age. Select the most likely cause:*

A Respiratory distress syndrome

B Transient tachypnoea of the newborn

C Group B streptococcal infection

D Meconium aspiration

E Pneumothorax

11.

i) What is this condition?

ii) What is the management?

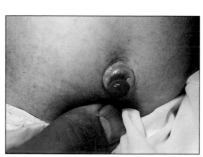

Fig. 9.11

9. i)

ii) A B C D E

iii) A B C D E

10. A B C D E

11. i)

   ii)

1. A *False.* Preterm is defined as less than 37 weeks' gestation.
    B *True.* Low birthweight is less than 2.5 kg, irrespective of gestational age.
    C *False.* The neonatal mortality is the number of neonatal deaths in the first four weeks (i.e. less than 28 days old) per 1000 live births.
    D *False.* An infant born with any signs of life but dying shortly afterwards is classified as a neonatal death.
    E *True.*

2. A *False.* Most infants with a low Apgar score at one minute have not experienced birth asphyxia and recover quickly.
    B *True.*
    C *True.*
    D *False.* Recurrent seizures are a feature of moderate or severe hypoxic ischaemic encephalopathy.
    E *False.* Birth asphyxia is responsible for only 10–15% of cerebral palsy. In most cases of cerebral palsy no cause is identified.

3. Fig. 9.1   Chignon
    Fig. 9.2   Cephalhaematoma
    Fig. 9.3   Forceps mark
    Fig. 9.4   Fractured left clavicle

4. A *True.* The Dubowitz examination is an example.
    B *False.* Surfactant reduces surface tension.
    C *True.*
    D *False.* Infants only suck and swallow milk at 35–36 weeks' gestation.
    E *True.*

5. i)   Diffuse granular or 'ground glass' appearance of lung fields.
         Air bronchogram (an outline of the air filled bronchi against poorly aerated lung)
    ii) **D**. Respiratory distress syndrome.
    iii) Asymmetrical chest movement
         Decreased air entry on affected side
         Deviated trachea/apex
         Translucency on cold light examination
    iv) Left. There is hyperlucency on the left, the lung edge on the left is visible and the mediastinum is displaced to the right.
    v)

		Day 5	Day 15
A	Normal		
B	Intraventricular haemorrhage	✓	
C	Subdural haemorrhage		
D	Ventricular dilatation		✓
E	Periventricular leucomalacia		

6. Bronchopulmonary dysplasia (chronic lung disease of prematurity).

7. The right arm is preductal, the left arm post-ductal and may record a lower oxygen tension if there is shunting of deoxygenated blood through the duct from the pulmonary artery into the aorta.

8. i)   Jaundice within the first 24 hours may progress rapidly and requires aggressive management.
    ii) Full blood count and film
         Blood group of infant
         Direct antiglobulin (Coombs) test
         Determine mother's blood group

iii) **B**: haemolysis. The very rapid rise in bilirubin is characteristic of haemolysis, e.g. ABO incompatibility or Rhesus disease.
Physiological and breast-milk jaundice do not occur in the first day of life.
Biliary atresia causes prolonged, conjugated jaundice.
Congenital hypothyroidism causes a mild, unconjugated jaundice.
iv) Hearing.

9. i) Is the baby well? Jaundice can be a sign of illness, especially sepsis.
Is the jaundice marked? Otherwise it is unlikely to be clinically significant. However, assessment of jaundice is notoriously unreliable in black babies.
What is mother's blood group and antibody status during pregnancy? This will alert you to a potential haemolytic cause.
Jaundice in previous children? ABO incompatibility may recur.
Is she breastfed? Breastfeeding may exacerbate physiological jaundice.
ii) **C**. Physiological.
Sickle cell disease does not cause neonatal jaundice.
Rhesus incompatibility usually presents within the first 24 hours of life.
Hypothyroidism is uncommon and causes a mild but prolonged jaundice.
Biliary atresia causes prolonged, conjugated jaundice.
iii) **E**. This is a low level of jaundice and at three days of age is most likely to resolve spontaneously.
Further assessment is required if it becomes more severe or if it has not resolved by 14 days of age.

10. **B**. Transient tachypnoea of the newborn is the commonest cause of respiratory distress in a term infant. It especially occurs following caesarean section.
Respiratory distress syndrome is rare in term infants.
Group B streptococcal infection is uncommon following an elective caesarean section, but must always be considered in any baby with respiratory distress.
Meconium aspiration is usually symptomatic from birth. Symptomatic pneumothorax in the absence of lung disease is uncommon.

11. i) Umbilical granuloma
ii) Apply silver nitrate / remove surgically

10 Growth and puberty

1. *Which of the following statements about growth are true or false:*

A In infancy it is predominantly dependent on nutrition rather than growth hormone.

B Growth of the long bones ceases with epiphyseal fusion

C Bone age is used to assess skeletal maturation

D In females the growth spurt occurs after the menarche

E Females have a greater pubertal growth spurt

2. *Which of the following statements about puberty are true or false:*

A Breast development is the first sign in females

B Penile growth is the first sign in males

C A nine-year-old boy would be expected to have some axillary and pubic hair

D A testicular volume of 2 ml is prepubertal

E Some breast development may occur in normal pubertal males

3. *These figures show pubertal changes.*

i) Select the appropriate staging of female breast changes (Fig. 10.1):

BI   Prepubertal
BII   Breast bud
BIII   Juvenile smooth contour
BIV   Areola and papilla project above
        the breast
V   Adult

ii) Select the appropriate stage of male genital changes (Fig. 10.2):

GI   Pre-adolescent
GII   Enlargement of testes and
        scrotum, change in texture of
        scrotum, but little penile
        enlargement

GIII   Growth in length and
        circumference of penis, with
        further testicular and scrotal
        growth

GIV   Increased size of penis and
        development of glans,
        enlargement of testes and
        scrotum and darkening of
        scrotal skin

GV   Adult genitalia

1.
A True ❏   False ❏
B True ❏   False ❏
C True ❏   False ❏
D True ❏   False ❏
E True ❏   False ❏

2.
A True ❏   False ❏
B True ❏   False ❏
C True ❏   False ❏
D True ❏   False ❏
E True ❏   False ❏

3. i) B I II III IV V
    ii) G I II III IV V

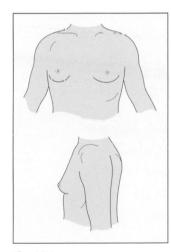

Fig. 10.1

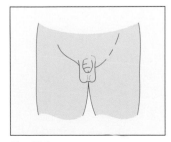

Fig. 10.2

iii) Select the appropriate stage in pubic hair changes (Fig. 10.3):

PHI   Pre-adolescent

PHII Sparse, pigmented, long, straight, mainly along labia

PHIII Darker, coarser, curlier and more widespread

PHIV Adult in nature, but less extensive distribution

PHV   Adult

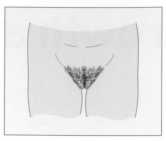

Fig. 10.3

iii) PH I II III IV V

4. *Abdulla (date of birth 10 June 1995) was seen because of parental concern about his short stature.*

Date	Weight	Height
10.6.95	3.3 kg	54 cm
21.11.97	10.9 kg	85 cm
31.9.98	11.8 kg	91 cm
7.6.99	14.9 kg	94 cm

i)   Plot the data on the growth chart (Fig. 10.4).

ii) What information can be gained from measuring the height of both parents?

iii) Mother's height is 152 cm (2nd centile) and father's height is 172 cm (25th centile). Select the most likely cause of his short stature:

A   Growth hormone deficiency

B   Familial short stature

C   Hypothyroidism

D   Turner's syndrome

E   Achondroplasia

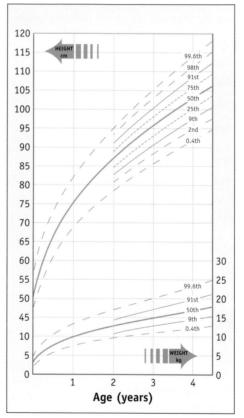

Fig. 10.4 (based on chart © Child Growth Foundation)

4.

ii)

iii)   A B C D E

5. *Evelyn (Fig. 10.5), aged eight years, is referred to outpatients by her general practitioner. Her mother is concerned that she is smaller than her six-year-old sister. She is in good health.*

   i) What single investigation would you perform?

   ii) What is the most likely diagnosis?

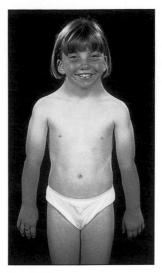

Fig. 10.5

5. i)

   ii)

6. *Peter, aged six years, is assessed in outpatients because of concern about his short stature. Examination is otherwise normal. His growth chart is shown in Fig. 10.6. Growth hormone deficiency is suspected.*

   Select the most appropriate diagnostic test:

   A Short synacthen test

   B Growth hormone provocation test

   C Early morning growth hormone assay

   D Ultrasound of his adrenal glands

   E Skull X-ray

6. A B C D E

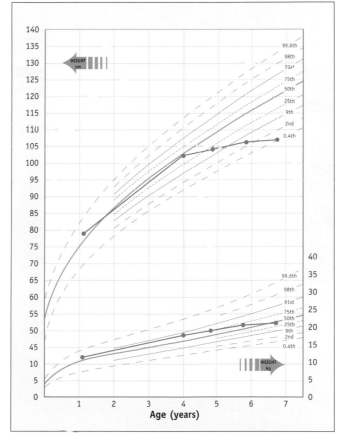

Fig. 10.6 (based on chart © Child Growth Foundation)

7. *Darren, aged 14, is concerned because he is much shorter than his classmates. He is well but is frustrated at being unable to get into any of the school sports teams. His father reveals that he was also short as a child but is now of average height. Darren's examination is normal. He has no pubic hair, his testes are 3 ml and his penis is pre-adolescent. His bone age is 12 years. His growth chart is shown in Fig. 10.7.*

7. i)   A B C D E

ii)

i)   Select the most likely cause of his short stature:

   A   Hypothyroidism

   B   Cushing's syndrome

   C   Kleinfelter's syndrome

   D   Constitutional delay of growth and puberty

   E   Growth hormone deficiency

ii) What is his prognosis?

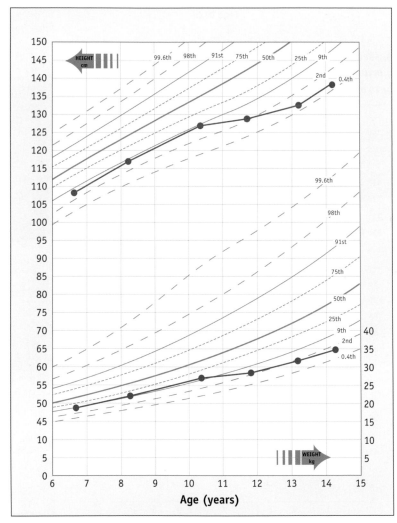

Fig. 10.7 (based on chart © Child Growth Foundation)

8. *John, aged three years, is referred to outpatients because of concern about the development of pubic and axillary hair. His testes are 1.5 ml in size (prepubertal). His blood pressure is 100/75. Gonadotrophin levels are normal for a prepubertal boy but his bone age is five years.*

   Select the most likely cause of his early pubertal development:

   A   Adrenal tumour

   B   Brain tumour

   C   Familial precocious puberty

   D   Testicular tumour

   E   Prader–Willi syndrome

8. A B C D E

9. *George, aged two weeks, presents with vomiting, diarrhoea and poor feeding. Investigations show:*

   Sodium 112 mmol/l (normal range 133–145 mmol/l)

   Potassium 6.2 mmol/l (normal range 3.5–6.0 mmol/l)

   Urea 7.8 mmol/l (normal range 2.5–8.0 mmol/l)

   Creatinine 30 (μmol/l (normal range 20–65 (mol/l)

   Blood glucose 2 mmol/l

   Infection screen – negative

   i)   What is the most likely diagnosis?

   A   Hypothyroidism

   B   Cushing's syndrome

   C   Inadequate sodium intake

   D   Congenital adrenal hyperplasia

   E   Acute renal failure

   ii) How may a female infant with this disorder present at birth?

   iii) What long-term drug treatment will George require? List two drugs.

9. i) A B C D E
   ii)

   iii)

10. *Fig. 10.8*

   i)   What is this condition called?

   ii) What would you tell the child's parents at birth?

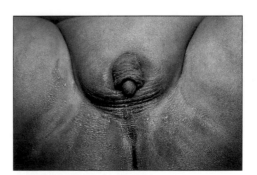

Fig. 10.8

10. i)

   ii)

1. **A** *True.*
   B *True.* However, some small increase in height may still occur because of growth of the spine.
   C *True.*
   D *False.* Only 4% of final height growth occurs after menarche.
   E *False.* Males have a greater pubertal growth spurt.

2. **A** *True.*
   B *False.* Increase in testicular volume is the first sign of puberty in males.
   C *False.* You would expect a nine-year-old boy to be prepubertal.
   D *True.*
   E *True.*

3. i) BIII
   ii) GII
   iii) PHII

4. i)

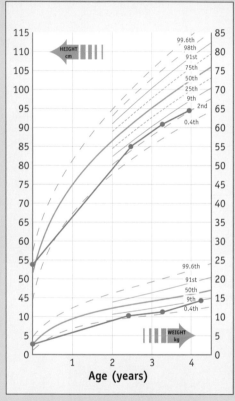

Fig. 10.9 (based in chart © Child Growth Foundation)

   ii) The mid-parental height is a guide to the child's genetic growth potential. It is calculated using a standard formula.
   iii) **B**. Familial short stature. He is growing consistently along the 2nd centile for height. This is in keeping with his mid-parental height.

   In hypothyroidism and growth hormone deficiency, the growth rate is markedly reduced and affected children fall off their height centile. Turner's syndrome only affects females and children with achondroplasia are much shorter than this child.

5. i) Karyotype.
   ii) Turner's syndrome.

6. **B.** A pituitary provocation test using clonidine, glucagon or insulin is required.

7. i) **D.** Constitutional delay of growth and puberty.
    ii)   Good. He should eventually achieve a height corresponding to his mid-parental height. Delay in his skeletal maturation means that he will on average continue to grow for two years more than his peers.

8. **A.** As his testes are prepubertal, the advanced development of pubic and axillary hair and advanced bone age must be the result of androgen production elsewhere, usually the adrenal gland. He does not have true precocious puberty as his testes are small.

9. i)   **D.** Congenital adrenal hyperplasia. The combination of hyponatraemia, hyperkalaemia and hypoglycaemia are suggestive of glucocorticoid deficiency. Hyponatraemia may be a feature of acute renal failure, but this child has a normal plasma urea and creatinine.
    ii)   Virilisation of the external genitalia.
    iii) Mineralocorticoid replacement therapy, as fludrocortisone.
          Glucocorticoid replacement therapy, e.g. hydrocortisone.

10. i)   Ambiguous genitalia.
    ii)   We are unable to determine whether the baby is female or male until further investigations have been performed. We will then be able to assign the baby's sex appropriately. Until then the baby's birth should not be registered.

11 Nutrition

1. *The following are advantages of breast compared with formula feeding:*

A   A lower incidence of gastrointestinal infection.

B   A reduced incidence of haemorrhagic disease of the newborn.

C   A reduced incidence of neonatal jaundice.

D   Protection against the transmission of maternal HIV infection.

E   Reliable form of contraception.

1.

A   True ☐   False ☐

B   True ☐   False ☐

C   True ☐   False ☐

D   True ☐   False ☐

E   True ☐   False ☐

2. *Complete the table below comparing the composition of breast and unmodified cow's (doorstep) milk*

	Breast milk	Cow's milk
A Higher concentration of calcium		
B Higher concentration of phosphorus		
C Iron more bio-available		
D Higher concentration of sodium		
E Protein predominantly casein		

3. *What is meant by the term 'failure to thrive'?*

3.

4. *The mother of Amy, aged 11 months, complains that her daughter eats very little. Her growth chart is shown (Fig. 11.1). She tries to force her to eat more but this causes crying and occasional vomiting. Amy is otherwise well and her development is normal.*

i)   Is Amy failing to thrive?

ii) What is the most likely explanation for Amy's low weight?

iii) What advice would you give regarding Amy's poor appetite?

iv) How could you check your diagnosis is correct?

4. i) Yes ❑   No ❑

ii)

iii)

iv)

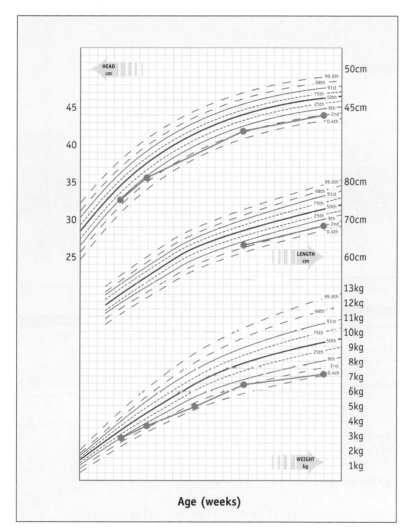

Fig. 11.1 (based on chart © Child Growth Foundation)

5. *David, aged 2½ years, is referred because of poor weight gain. He has had two recent admissions with chest infections requiring intravenous antibiotics. This is his growth chart from his personal child health record (Fig. 11.2).*

i) List two further questions which would help in establishing the most likely diagnosis.

ii) What is the most likely diagnosis?

iii) Although his appetite is good and he eats a well-balanced diet he is failing to thrive. Give one reason for this.

5. i)

ii)

iii)

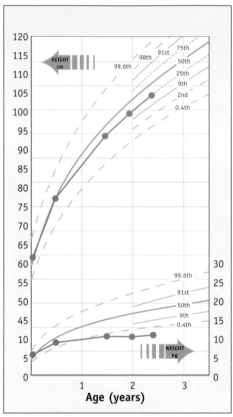

Fig. 11.2 (based on chart © Child Growth Foundation)

6.

7.

6. *Why might an infant fail to thrive in the absence of an identified organic cause?*

7. *Complete the table below about marasmus and kwashiorkor by placing a tick in the appropriate box. Some features may apply to both.*

	Clinical feature	Marasmus	Kwashiorkor
A	< 60% expected body weight		
B	Oedema		
C	Muscle wasting		
D	Sparse, depigmented hair		
E	Distended abdomen and enlarged liver		

8. *Babatunde, a 13-month-old Black African boy, presents with a brief generalised convulsion. He has not been febrile or unwell. He is still entirely breastfed. His wrists are noted to be swollen.*

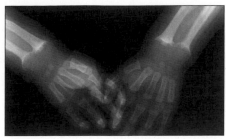

Fig. 11.3

i) His wrist X-ray is shown in Fig. 11.3. List two abnormalities.

ii) What is the radiological diagnosis?

iii) Which of the three patterns of biochemical results would you expect?

	Calcium	Phosphate	Alkaline phosphatase
A	Low	High	Mildly raised
B	Low/normal	Low	Markedly raised
C	Normal	Normal	Normal

iv) What is the most likely cause?

v) What two management steps are required?

9. *What is the role of sunlight in vitamin D metabolism?*

10. *List two organic causes of obesity.*

8. i)

   ii)

   iii) A   B   C

   iv)

   v)

9.

10.

1. **A** *True.*
   B *False.* Breast milk is deficient in vitamin K.
   C *False.*
   D *False.* Breastfeeding increases the risk of transmission to the baby.
   E *False.* However, on a population basis, it increases the time interval between children and so reduces the overall birth rate.

2.

		Breast milk	Cow's milk
A	Higher concentration of calcium		✓
B	Higher concentration of phosphorus		✓
C	Iron more bio-available	✓	
D	Higher concentration of sodium		✓
E	Protein predominantly casein		✓

3. Failure to thrive is suboptimal weight gain/growth in infants and young children. It is demonstrated by serial growth measurements showing a fall across two or more centile lines.

4. i) No.
   ii) She is a normal, short and slim girl.
   iii) A nutritionally balanced, mixed diet should be offered in a non-confrontational way. Infants often graze, eating little and often rather than formal meals.
   iv) Monitor her growth to show that she maintains her present centiles.

5. i) Has he had gastrointestinal problems; in particular, are his stools abnormal?
   Is there a relevant family history?
   What is his dietary intake?
   ii) Cystic fibrosis.
   iii) Malabsorption due to pancreatic insufficiency.
   Increased energy requirement mainly because of chronic respiratory infection.

6. Environmental deprivation (so-called non-organic failure to thrive). This may be because of maternal psychiatric illness, parental learning difficulties or other adverse social circumstances.

7.

	Clinical feature	Marasmus	Kwashiorkor
A	< 60% expected body weight	✓	
B	Oedema		✓
C	Muscle wasting	✓	✓
D	Sparse, depigmented hair		✓
E	Distended abdomen and enlarged liver		✓

8. i) Ends of the radius and ulna expanded, rarefied and cup-shaped.
   Poorly mineralised bones.
   ii) Rickets.
   iii) **B.**
   iv) Nutritional vitamin D deficiency from prolonged, exclusive breastfeeding.
   v) Introduction of solid food.
   Oral vitamin D supplementation.

9. It forms vitamin D_3 in the skin from cholesterol.

10. Cushing's syndrome
    Hypothyroidism
    Syndrome associated with obesity, e.g. Prader–Willi
    Almost all cases of obesity in children are, however, non-organic and related to excessive food intake relative to exercise.

12 Gastroenterology

1. *The following are case histories of children presenting with vomiting. Match each history with the most likely diagnosis by ticking the appropriate box in the table below.*

   A A four-hour-old infant vomiting bile

   B A five-day-old term infant is vomiting, not feeding and is increasingly lethargic. His temperature is 35.5°C

   C A five-week-old male infant who has forcefully vomited after almost every feed in the last 36 hours but continues to take his milk well

   D A one-year-old boy who is just recovering from an upper respiratory tract infection and develops paroxysmal episodes of abdominal pain and pallor associated with vomiting

   E An eight-year-old girl who presents with vomiting and abdominal pain and has rapid, deep breathing

Case history	Diagnosis				
	Diabetic ketoacidosis	Intussusception	Malrotation	Pyloric stenosis	Septicaemia
A					
B					
C					
D					
E					

2. *Which of the following statements about gastro-oesophageal reflux are true or false:*

   A It characteristically resolves spontaneously by one year of age

   B It should only be treated if associated with failure to thrive

   C It is a cause of iron deficiency anaemia

   D Preterm infants are at increased risk

   E The oesophageal pH trace shown confirms the diagnosis (Fig. 12.1)

2.

A True ❑   False ❑
B True ❑   False ❑
C True ❑   False ❑
D True ❑   False ❑
E True ❑   False ❑

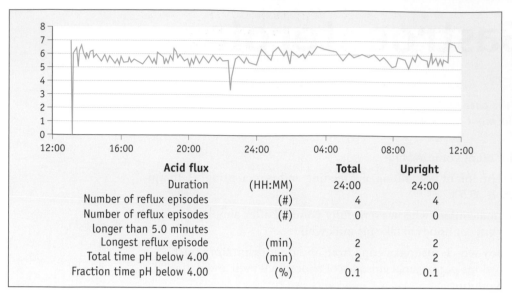

Acid flux		Total	Upright
Duration	(HH:MM)	24:00	24:00
Number of reflux episodes	(#)	4	4
Number of reflux episodes longer than 5.0 minutes	(#)	0	0
Longest reflux episode	(min)	2	2
Total time pH below 4.00	(min)	2	2
Fraction time pH below 4.00	(%)	0.1	0.1

Fig. 12.1

3. *Which of the following statements about pyloric stenosis are true or false:*

A A positive family history places the infant at increased risk

B The vomiting is bile-stained

C During a positive test feed a mass is palpable in the right upper quadrant of the abdomen

D Hyperchloraemic alkalosis is characteristic

E The immediate management is surgical

3.

A True ❏ False ❏

B True ❏ False ❏

C True ❏ False ❏

D True ❏ False ❏

E True ❏ False ❏

4. *Max, aged two years, has had a two-day history of fever and coryza. His mother has brought him to the Accident and Emergency Department as he is crying inconsolably. She thinks that his tummy is hurting him. Given each of the following examination findings, what is the most likely cause of his abdominal pain?*

A His throat is red and he has tender cervical lymph nodes, mild generalised tenderness of the abdomen with no guarding.

B He looks pale and has a pulse of 180/min, cool peripheries and a mass in the right upper quadrant. He has just vomited.

C He is sitting quietly on his mother's lap, is reluctant to play, has a respiratory rate of 50/min and reduced breath sounds at the right base.

D He appears unwell with diffuse abdominal tenderness and a small lump in the right inguinal region.

E He appears reasonably well with minimal abdominal tenderness but has an indentable mass on the left side of the abdomen.

4. A

B

C

D

E

5. *Molly, aged six years, has had vomiting and central abdominal pain for two days. She develops diarrhoea. Examination reveals mild dehydration, fever of 38°C, tachycardia of 110/min and tenderness in the lower right abdomen with no guarding or rebound tenderness.*

i) Complete the table below giving one likely diagnosis for each of the following urine dipstick findings.

Dipstick	Diagnosis
Glucose++++ and ketones (large)	
Leucocytes++	
Bilirubin+++	
Protein++++	
Blood+++	

In fact, Molly's urine dipstick and microscopy were normal. When asked to walk, she is unable to stand up straight because of pain.

ii) Select the most likely diagnosis:

A Mesenteric adenitis

B Acute appendicitis

C Slipped disc

D Urinary tract infection

E Psychosomatic

5. ii) A B C D E

6. *Which of the following statements about recurrent abdominal pain of childhood are true or false:*

A The pain is characteristically periumbilical

B Urine microscopy and culture should be performed

C If accompanied by weight loss, inflammatory bowel disease needs to be excluded

D A psychological cause can usually be identified

E The pain characteristically wakes the child during the night

6.

A True ❏ False ❏

B True ❏ False ❏

C True ❏ False ❏

D True ❏ False ❏

E True ❏ False ❏

7. *This photograph (Fig. 12.2) was taken shortly after the skin had been pinched. What physical sign is shown?*

7.

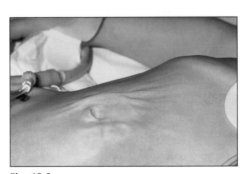

Fig. 12.2

8. *Joshua, aged six months, has had a three-day history of diarrhoea and vomiting. During the last 24 hours he has been feeding poorly and has had fewer wet nappies than usual. On examination he is found to be quiet but alert, has a tachycardia, reduced skin turgor, sunken fontanelle, dry mouth and is tachypnoeic. The capillary refill time is normal. His blood pressure is normal for his age.*

i) How dehydrated is Joshua?

ii) His plasma sodium is found to be 156 mmol/l (normal range 135–145 mmol/l). How does the hypernatraemia affect his management?

9. *This is a diagrammatic representation of the intracellular (ICC) and extracellular (ECC) fluid compartments (Fig. 12.3). When a child becomes dehydrated, water moves between the intracellular and extracellular compartments.*

Place an arrowhead on the blue line to indicate the direction that water moves in hypernatraemic and hyponatraemic dehydration.

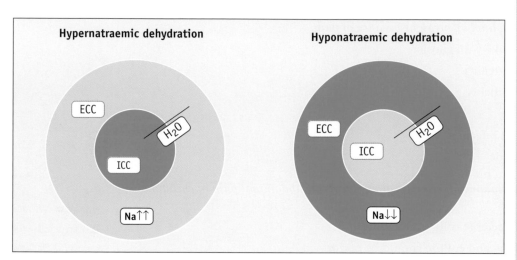

Fig. 12.3

10. *Complete the table below selecting:*

i) the commonest cause of gastroenteritis in developed countries

ii) one or more organisms causing bloody diarrhoea.

Organism	Commonest cause of gastroenteritis in developed countries	Bloody diarrhoea
Salmonella		
Shigella		
Rotavirus		
Campylobacter jejuni		
E. Coli		

11. *In developing countries, oral rehydration solutions save millions of lives. What is the role of glucose or sucrose in these solutions?*

12. *Jenny, aged 14 months, develops gastroenteritis which responds to oral glucose electrolyte solution. However, the diarrhoea reoccurs on introducing a normal diet. Give one likely cause (other than continuing infection).*

8. i)

   ii)

11.

12.

13. *Which of the following are characteristic features of coeliac disease:*

A   Irritability

B   Iron deficiency anaemia

C   Recurrent urticaria

D   Growth failure

E   An increased risk of small bowel lymphoma

14. *Rodney, a boisterous two-year-old, has had diarrhoea for the last three months. He produces up to four stools a day which are very loose, brown in colour and usually contain undigested carrots and other food. The rest of the family are well. He has never been abroad. Examination is normal and his personal child health record shows that he is growing along the 50th centile for weight and 75th centile for height.*

What is the likely cause of his diarrhoea?

15. *Which of the following statements about constipation are true or false:*

A   Hirschsprung's disease characteristically commences in the second year of life

B   It is a cause of abdominal pain in children

C   Diarrhoea is a recognised presenting feature

D   It is a recognised side effect of codeine treatment

E   It is a clinical feature of hyperthyroidism

13.

A   True ❑   False ❑

B   True ❑   False ❑

C   True ❑   False ❑

D   True ❑   False ❑

E   True ❑   False ❑

14.

15.

A   True ❑   False ❑

B   True ❑   False ❑

C   True ❑   False ❑

D   True ❑   False ❑

E   True ❑   False ❑

1. Case history

	Diabetic ketoacidosis	Intussusception	Malrotation	Pyloric stenosis	Septicaemia
A			✓		
B					✓
C				✓	
D		✓			
E	✓				

Comments:
A   Malrotation must be excluded in any newborn infant who vomits bile.
B   An infant who is unwell, has temperature instability and vomiting may be septicaemic.
C   In pyloric stenosis the vomiting is characteristically forceful but initially the child is well.
D   This is the characteristic history of intussusception.
E   Diabetic ketoacidosis may mimic an acute abdomen. The rapid deep breathing is Kussmaul breathing from acidosis.

2.   A   *True.*
    B   *False.* Other indications are repeated regurgitation, apnoea and aspiration.
    C   *True.* This is a result of reduced intake from vomiting and / or bleeding from oesophagitis.
    D   *True.*
    E   *False.* The oesophageal pH trace shown is normal as the pH is below 4 only infrequently.

3.   A   *True.*
    B   *False.* The obstruction is above the entry point of the common bile duct (Ampulla of Vater) and the vomit will not contain bile.
    C   *True.*
    D   *False.* There is a hypochloraemic alkalosis from vomiting stomach contents containing hydrochloric acid.
    E   *False.* The immediate management priority is to correct any fluid and electrolyte abnormalities prior to surgery.

4.   A   Mesenteric adenitis
    B   Intussusception
    C   Right lower lobe pneumonia
    D   Right strangulated inguinal hernia
    E   Constipation

5.   i)

Dipstick	Diagnosis
Glucose++++ and ketones (large)	Diabetic ketoacidosis
Leucocytes++	Urinary tract infection
Bilirubin+++	Hepatitis
Protein++++	Nephrotic syndrome
Blood+++	Nephritis, urinary tract infection

ii)   **B.** The inability to stand up straight because of pain is known as the 'appendix shuffle' and is adopted to minimise the painful movement of inflamed adjacent peritoneal surfaces. Appendicitis is the commonest cause in children.

6. **A** *True.*
    B *True.*
    C *True.*
    D *False.* Although stress sometimes causes psychosomatic symptoms, in the majority no specific psychological cause is identified.
    E *False.*

7. Reduced skin turgor. It may be caused by dehydration or malnutrition.

8. i) 5–10%, that is, moderate dehydration. If severe (>10%) he would have been drowsy, peripherally cold, capillary refill time would have been prolonged and his urine output markedly reduced.
    ii) His rehydration should be slow to avoid the risk of convulsions associated with rapid osmotic shift. However, if in shock, this must first be rapidly corrected.

9.

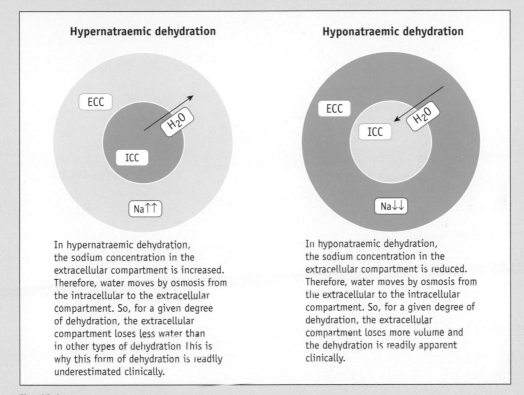

Hypernatraemic dehydration

ECC

H_2O

ICC

Na$\uparrow\uparrow$

In hypernatraemic dehydration, the sodium concentration in the extracellular compartment is increased. Therefore, water moves by osmosis from the intracellular to the extracellular compartment. So, for a given degree of dehydration, the extracellular compartment loses less water than in other types of dehydration This is why this form of dehydration is readily underestimated clinically.

Hyponatraemic dehydration

ECC

ICC

H_2O

Na$\downarrow\downarrow$

In hyponatraemic dehydration, the sodium concentration in the extracellular compartment is reduced. Therefore, water moves by osmosis from the extracellular to the intracellular compartment. So, for a given degree of dehydration, the extracellular compartment loses more volume and the dehydration is readily apparent clinically.

Fig. 12.4

10.

Organism	Commonest cause of gastroenteritis in developed countries	Bloody diarrhoea
Salmonella		✓
Shigella		✓
Rotavirus	✓	
Campylobacter jejuni		✓
E. Coli		✓

11. They enhance sodium and water absorption from the bowel.

12. Transient lactose intolerance.

    Cow's milk protein intolerance.

13. A *True.*
    B *True.*
    C *False.*
    D *True.*
    E *True.* This occurs in adult life.

14. Toddler diarrhoea.

15. A *False.* It characteristically presents in the neonatal period or early infancy.
    B *True.*
    C *True.* Overflow diarrhoea – leakage of liquid stool around impacted faeces.
    D *True.*
    E *False.* It is a feature of hypothyroidism.

13 Infection and immunity

1. *Harry, aged 21 months, presents with a three-day history of cough and fever. Examination reveals conjunctivitis and this widespread rash (Fig. 13.1). You suspect he may have measles.*

i) What pathognomic sign would you look for?

ii) List two complications he might develop during this febrile illness.

iii) Name one late complication.

iv) Which oral supplement improves the outcome of measles in developing countries?

v) Should Harry be separated from his three-year-old sister to prevent her catching the infection?

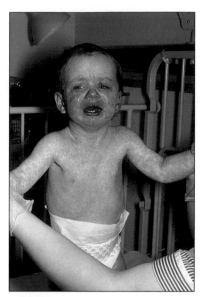

Fig. 13.1

1. i)

   ii)

   iii)

   iv)

   v) Yes ❑ No ❑

2. *Ella, aged three, has been unwell for 24 hours with irritability, vomiting and fever. She was seen by her general practitioner earlier in the day and started on amoxycillin. On examination her temperature is 38.5°C, pulse 140/min and blood pressure 90/60. The rash on her limbs and upper chest is shown (Fig. 13.2). Some of the lesions do not blanch on finger pressure. Her hands and feet feel cold and her capillary refill time is 5 sec. She watches attentively, and talks to her mother. There is no neck stiffness and Kernig's sign is negative.*

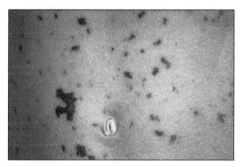

Fig. 13.2

i) How would you describe the skin lesions?

ii) Which of the following statements are true or false:

   A Meningitis is the most likely diagnosis

   B Kernig's sign is positive if there is back pain on extension of the knee with the hips held flexed

   C The most likely organism causing her illness is *Haemophilus influenzae* type b

   D Her negative blood culture excludes a bacterial infection

   E A lumbar puncture is urgently indicated

2.

i)

ii)
   A True ❑ False ❑
   B True ❑ False ❑
   C True ❑ False ❑
   D True ❑ False ❑
   E True ❑ False ❑

iii) A B C D E

iii) Select her most pressing clinical problem:

   A Raised intracranial pressure

   B A generalised coagulation disorder

   C Fever

   D Tachycardia

   E Septic shock

3. *In the investigation of a child with suspected meningitis, CSF is sent for urgent microscopy and biochemical analysis. Complete the table below by placing a tick indicating the most likely diagnosis.*

CSF microscopy	CSF Protein g/l	CSF Glucose mmol/l	Blood Glucose mmol/l	Diagnosis			
				Viral	Bacterial	Blood-stained tap	TB
A 1500 neutrophils	0.6	2.1	7.2				
B 125 lymphocytes 12 neutrophils	0.3	4.1	5.6				
C 95 lymphocytes 10 neutrophils	2.2	1.2	6.3				
D 2 lymphocytes 4200 red blood cells	0.3	3.4	5.3				

Normal CSF values: Microscopy WBC 0–5 mm³, RBC 0 mm³, Protein 0.15–0.4 g/l, Glucose > 50% of blood glucose

4. *Which of the following statements about common childhood infections are true or false:*

A Mumps is unlikely if the parotid swelling and earache are unilateral

B Bilateral parotid enlargement is characteristic of both mumps and HIV infection

C Gingivostomatitis is caused by recurrent HSV infection

D Human herpes virus 6 (HHV6) is a cause of febrile convulsions

E Ataxia is a characteristic feature of chicken pox encephalitis

4.

A True ❑ False ❑

B True ❑ False ❑

C True ❑ False ❑

D True ❑ False ❑

E True ❑ False ❑

5. i)

   ii)

5. *Jennifer, aged nine years, developed a severe sore throat and lethargy. Tonsillitis was diagnosed, a throat swab taken, and amoxycillin prescribed. Two days later she develops this florid maculopapular rash (Fig. 13.3).*

i) What is the most likely cause of her sore throat?

ii) Why has she developed this rash?

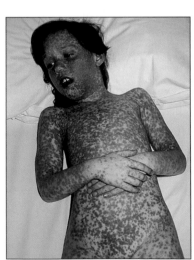

Fig. 13.3

6. *What common infections are shown?*

i) **Fig. 13.4**

ii) **Fig. 13.5** a and b

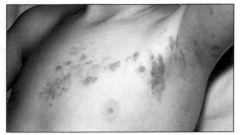

Fig. 13.4

6. i)

   ii)

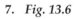

Fig. 13.5a   Fig. 13.5b

7. *Fig. 13.6*

i) What is this condition?
ii) List two potential complications.

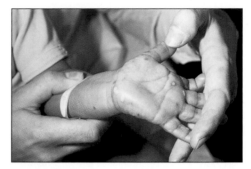

Fig. 13.6

7. i)

   ii)

8. *This boy has Kawasaki's disease.*

i) What abnormality is shown (Fig. 13.7)?

ii) List two other diagnostic clinical features.

iii) What serious complication may occur?

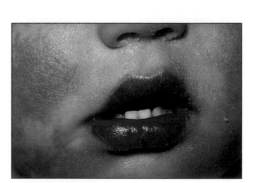

Fig. 13.7

8. i)

   ii)

   iii)

9. *Imran, aged three years, moved to the UK from Bangladesh four months ago. He has had a poor appetite, little weight gain and a cough for several months. His general practitioner requests a chest X-ray (Fig. 13.8).*

   i) What is the most likely diagnosis?

   ii) What is the likely infective source in this child?

   iii) What public health measures should be initiated?

   iv) List two reasons for the resurgence of this disease in the UK.

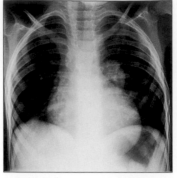

Fig. 13.8

9. i)

   ii)

   iii)

   iv)

10. *Sebastian, aged 10 years, has recently returned from a safari holiday in Kenya. He has had a fever for four days associated with rigors. This is his blood film (Fig. 13.9).*

    What is the diagnosis?

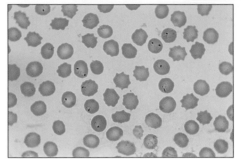

Fig. 13.9

10.

11. *Which of the following statements about immune function are true or false:*

A An infant has a lower total IgG than an adult

B Infants are more prone to viral infections at age 0–3 months than when 9–12 months old

C A toddler with four viral upper respiratory tract infections in the previous 12 months probably has an immune deficiency

D Splenectomy is associated with an increased risk of pneumococcal infection

E Defects in phagocytic function result in recurrent bacterial infections

11.

A True ❏ False ❏

B True ❏ False ❏

C True ❏ False ❏

D True ❏ False ❏

E True ❏ False ❏

12. *Prince, a four-month-old Black-African boy, develops a fever, poor feeding and breathlessness. On examination he appears pale and has marked intercostal recession. His oxygen saturation in air is 72%. He is intubated and ventilated. His chest X-ray is shown (Fig. 13.10).*

    i) What is the most likely cause of his respiratory failure?

    ii) What is the most likely underlying diagnosis?

    iii) What prophylactic antibiotic would have reduced the risk of Prince's respiratory problem?

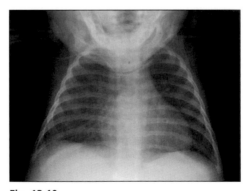

Fig. 13.10

12. i)

    ii)

    iii)

13. *Which of the following statements about HIV infection in children are true or false:*

A Transmission is usually from mother to child

B Diagnosis by detecting antibodies to HIV is unreliable in infancy

C Developmental regression is a feature of AIDS

D Breastfeeding reduces the transmission rate from mother to child

E There is no health advantage in diagnosing HIV infection in asymptomatic pregnant women

13.

A True ☐ False ☐

B True ☐ False ☐

C True ☐ False ☐

D True ☐ False ☐

E True ☐ False ☐

14. *Which of the following statements about immunisation are true or false:*

A The measles vaccine is inactivated

B BCG is a live attenuated vaccine

C A mild febrile illness is a contraindication to giving a vaccine

D Following a severe local reaction to a DPT vaccine, the next vaccination should be delayed for at least two months

E Eczema is a contraindication to MMR vaccine

14.

A True ☐ False ☐

B True ☐ False ☐

C True ☐ False ☐

D True ☐ False ☐

E True ☐ False ☐

15. *Peter, aged 18 months, has sustained a laceration whilst playing on his parents' farm. The wound requires suturing. His mother says that he has 'had all his vaccines'.*

i) Which vaccines should he have received and when?

ii) Does he need a tetanus booster?

15. i)

ii) Yes ☐ No ☐

1. i) Koplik spots – white spots on the buccal mucosa (Fig. 13.11).
   ii) Pneumonia
   Secondary bacterial infection and otitis media
   Tracheitis
   Febrile convulsion
   Uncommon complications are diarrhoea, hepatitis, appendicitis, myocarditis.
   iii) Encephalitis
   Subacute sclerosing panencephalitis (SSPE).
   iv) Vitamin A.
   v) No. He was already infectious for several days before he developed the rash.

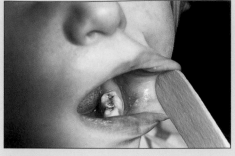

Fig. 13.11

2. i) Petechiae or purpura.
   ii) **A** *False.* There is no evidence of meningitis.
   B *True.*
   C *False.* The rash is characteristic of meningococcal disease. Hib vaccination has made infection with *Haemophilus influenzae* type B very uncommon.
   D *False.* Her blood cultures may well be negative as she has received oral antibiotics.
   E *False.* Lumbar puncture should be delayed until the child's condition is stable.
   iii) **E.** The priority in her management is the correction of shock.

3.

	CSF microscopy	CSF Protein g/l	CSF Glucose mmol/l	Blood Glucose mmol/l	Diagnosis			
					Viral	Bacterial	Blood-stained tap	TB
A	1500 neutrophils	0.6	2.1	7.2		✓		
B	125 lymphocytes 12 neutrophils	0.3	4.1	5.6	✓			
C	95 lymphocytes 10 neutrophils	2.2	1.2	6.3				✓
D	2 lymphocytes 4200 red blood cells	0.3	3.4	5.3			✓	

4. **A** *False.* Mumps can be unilateral.
   B *True.*
   C *False.* It is caused by a primary herpes simplex virus infection.
   D *True.*
   E *True.*

5. i) Epstein–Barr virus infection causing glandular fever (infectious mononucleosis).
   ii) Amoxycillin treatment of an EBV infection often results in a rash.

6. i) Varicella zoster (shingles).
   ii) Hand foot and mouth disease due to Coxsackie (an enterovirus) infection.

7. i) Periorbital cellulitis.
   ii) Direct spread of infection to the orbit
   Meningitis
   Cavernous sinus thrombosis.

8. i) Red, cracked lips (mucositis).
   ii) Fever of five or more days
       Conjunctival injection
       Mucous membrane changes – pharyngeal injection, strawberry tongue
       Cervical lymphadenopathy
       Rash (polymorphous)
       Red and oedematous palms and soles. Later peeling of the skin on the fingers and toes.
   iii) Coronary artery aneurysms.

9. i) Tuberculosis.
   ii) An infected adult in his household.
   iii) All household members should be screened with a tuberculin skin test and chest X-ray.
   iv) Immigration from countries of high prevalence
       Increased incidence in patients with HIV infection
       Emergence of multi-drug resistant strains.

10. *Falciparum* malaria.

11. A *True.*
    B *False.* In the first three months of life viral infections are uncommon because of passive transfer of protective maternal antibodies in the last trimester of pregnancy.
    C *False.*
    D *True.* There is also increased susceptibility to other encapsulated organisms such as *Haemophilus influenzae* and *Salmonella*.
    E *True.*

12. i) *Pneumocystis carinii* pneumonia.
    ii) Acquired immune deficiency syndrome (AIDS).
    iii) Cotrimoxazole.

13. A *True.*
    B *True.* Infants born to infected mothers will have circulating maternal HIV antibodies. The diagnosis is made by detecting virus in the infant's blood or by persistence of HIV antibodies after 18 months.
    C *True.*
    D *False.* Breastfeeding increases the transmission rate.
    E *False.* Anti-retroviral therapy for the mother and newborn infant, avoidance of breastfeeding and delivery by caesarean section have all been shown to substantially reduce the transmission rate.

14. A *False.* It is a live attenuated vaccine.
    B *True.*
    C *True.* A fever or systemic upset is a contraindication to immunisation.
    D *False.* This is an absolute contraindication to further doses of this vaccine.
    E *False.*

15. i) In the UK he should have received:
       DTP/Hib/Polio/Meningococcal C   2, 3 and 4 months
       MMR   12–18 months

    BCG may be given at birth, depending on local policy and if at increased risk
    DTP: Diphtheria, tetanus, pertussis
    Hib: *Haemophilus influenzae* type B
    Meningococcal C – since 1999 in UK
    MMR: Measles, mumps and rubella

    ii) No. He has received a full initial course of immunisation.

14 Respiratory disorders

1. *Liam, aged 10 years, complains of a sore throat and has a mild fever. The appearance of his throat is shown in Fig. 14.1.*

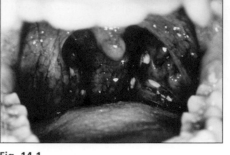

Fig. 14.1

   i) Select the most likely diagnosis:

   A Diphtheria

   B Acute epiglottitis

   C Exudative tonsillitis

   D Herpes simplex infection

   E Chicken pox

   ii) Name two common pathogens.

1. i) **A B C D E**
   ii)

2. *Jamal, aged 10 months, is brought at 1 a.m. to the Accident and Emergency department as he has woken up with noisy breathing. He has had a cold for two days and a barking cough for 12 hours. On examination he has a fever of 37.8°C and marked inspiratory stridor.*

   i) What is the most likely diagnosis?

   ii) List four treatment modalities available for this condition:

2. i)
   ii)

3. *This photograph (Fig. 14.2) was taken on intubating a child with severe stridor.*

   Select the single most likely diagnosis:

   A Foreign body

   B Quinsy

   C Retropharyngeal abscess

   D Epiglottitis

   E Nasal polyp

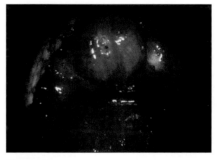

Fig. 14.2

3. **A B C D E**

4. i) What abnormality is shown in Fig. 14.3?
   ii) Give two likely causes.

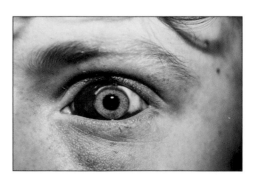

Fig. 14.3

4. i)

   ii)

5. *Amber, aged nine months, presents with a four-day history of coughing spasms which are followed by vomiting. Whooping cough (pertussis) is suspected. From the list below select how best to confirm the diagnosis:*

A By demonstrating a marked neutrophilia on a full blood count

B By demonstrating a marked lymphocytosis on a full blood count

C By immunofluorescence of a nasopharyngeal aspirate

D Culturing a pernasal swab

E By demonstrating patchy consolidation without collapse on a chest X-ray

6. *Jack, aged four months, is seen at home by his general practitioner because of two days of rapid, laboured breathing and poor feeding. He was born at 27 weeks' gestation, birth weight 979 g and was discharged home at three months of age. On examination he has a fever of 37.4°C and a respiratory rate of 60 breaths/min. His chest is hyperinflated with marked intercostal recession. On auscultation there are generalised fine crackles and wheezes.*

i) What is the most likely diagnosis?

ii) List two features which indicate that he should be admitted to hospital.

iii) On arrival at the Accident and Emergency department his oxygen saturation shows 88%. What is the initial management?

7. *Tak, aged three years, is taken to his general practitioner with a hacking cough. It started several weeks ago immediately after his birthday party and has failed to respond to two courses of antibiotics. He is otherwise well and has had no previous chest problems. On examination there is decreased air entry in the right lower zone with a normal percussion note.*

i) Which of the following statements are true or false:

A The chest signs are consistent with a pleural effusion

B A chest X-ray is indicated

C A therapeutic trial of an inhaled bronchodilator is indicated

D High dose oral antibiotics should be prescribed

E A sweat test should be obtained

ii) What is the most important diagnosis to consider?

5. A B C D E

6. i)

ii)

iii)

7. i)

A True ❑   False ❑

B True ❑   False ❑

C True ❑   False ❑

D True ❑   False ❑

E True ❑   False ❑

ii)

8. *Match each case history with the most appropriate chest X-ray by placing a tick in the appropriate column in the table below. For each case also give the most likely diagnosis.*

1 This eight-year-old child has had recurrent chest infections. His weight is on the 2nd centile and height on the 25th centile.

2 Four days ago this 10-year-old boy woke up during the night coughing and choking. Since then he has been noted to be intermittently wheezy.

3 This three-year-old girl has been coughing for 10 days with a fever and lethargy for two days.

4 During the last three weeks this four-month-old infant has fed poorly and developed increasingly laboured breathing.

A
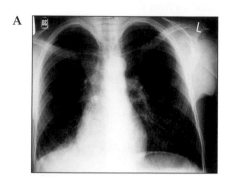
Fig. 14.4

B
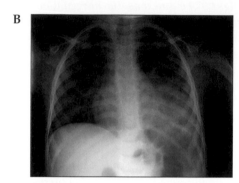
Fig. 14.5

C
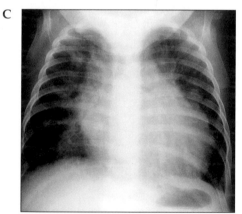
Fig. 14.6

D
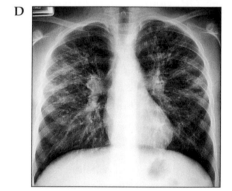
Fig. 14.7

Case history	Chest X-rays				Most likely diagnosis
	A	B	C	D	
1					
2					
3					
4					

9. *Which of the following statements about wheezing in children are true or false:*

A   Asthma in pre-school children is more commonly triggered by upper respiratory tract infections than exercise

B   Airway narrowing in asthma is caused only by smooth muscle contraction

C   A nocturnal cough without wheeze is a recognised presentation of asthma

D   Recurrent aspiration from gastro-oesophageal reflux is a recognised cause of wheeze

E   A peak flow in the normal range excludes the diagnosis of asthma

10. *In a three-year-old child with asthma select the single most effective mode of bronchodilator delivery from the list below:*

A   Metered dose inhaler (MDI) alone

B   Dry powder inhaler

C   Metered dose inhaler with spacer

D   Tablets

E   Syrup

11. *Sarah, aged 10 years, has frequent episodic asthma and presents to Accident and Emergency with increasing difficulty in breathing over the last 12 hours. Initial observation shows that she is anxious, sitting upright, has a marked tracheal tug and is unable to complete a sentence.*

i)   Which of the following statements are true or false:

   A   Her asthma attack is of moderate severity

   B   If there is no audible wheeze, this is reassuring

   C   Her condition is likely to improve if she is encouraged to lie flat

   D   Her oxygen saturation should be measured

   E   She should be taken promptly to the X-ray department for a chest X-ray

   There was minimal improvement with a salbutamol nebuliser and oxygen.

ii) Which of the following statements are true or false?

   A   A loading dose of aminophylline should now be given unless she is on regular theophylline

   B   An intravenous salbutamol infusion can be used as an alternative to aminophylline

   C   Intravenous hydrocortisone should be given

   D   No more than 28% of oxygen should be given

   E   A further dose of nebulised salbutamol should not be given for another four hours

12. *Zak, a three-year-old boy, is seen by his general practitioner because of recurrent wheezing associated with upper respiratory tract infections.*

   Which of the following features support the diagnosis of asthma?

A   Finger clubbing

B   Purulent sputum

C   A family history of asthma

D   Static weight for the last 12 months

E   The presence of eczema

9.
A   True ❑   False ❑
B   True ❑   False ❑
C   True ❑   False ❑
D   True ❑   False ❑
E   True ❑   False ❑

10.   A   B   C   D   E

11.
i)
A   True ❑   False ❑
B   True ❑   False ❑
C   True ❑   False ❑
D   True ❑   False ❑
E   True ❑   False ❑

ii)
A   True ❑   False ❑
B   True ❑   False ❑
C   True ❑   False ❑
D   True ❑   False ❑
E   True ❑   False ❑

12.
A   True ❑   False ❑
B   True ❑   False ❑
C   True ❑   False ❑
D   True ❑   False ❑
E   True ❑   False ❑

13. *Connor, a five-month-old boy visiting from Dublin, is admitted to hospital with respiratory distress and poor feeding. On examination he has a respiratory rate of 50 per minute with widespread crackles on auscultation of the chest. He was born at term with a birthweight of 3.6 kg (50th centile). His weight is now 5.2 kg (< 0.4th centile). He has never been a good feeder and has always tended to regurgitate. This is his first admission to hospital but he 'is always chesty'.*

i) List two clinical features from the history above which raise the possibility of cystic fibrosis.

ii) Which of these neonatal features in Connor's history would support the diagnosis of cystic fibrosis?

   A   Meconium aspiration

   B   Congenital pneumonia

   C   Delayed passage of meconium

   D   Hypoglycaemia

   E   Prolonged jaundice

iii) Cystic fibrosis is diagnosed. Which of the following does he require?

   A   A low-fat diet

   B   Regular chest percussion and postural drainage by his parents

   C   Vitamin C supplements

   D   Aggressive antibiotic treatment of chest infections

   E   Pancreatic enzyme supplements

14. *Which of the following statements about cystic fibrosis are true or false:*

A   The inheritance is autosomal recessive with a carrier rate in the UK of 1 in 25

B   There is a defect in transmembrane chloride transport

C   A chest X-ray is diagnostic restriction

D   It is associated with intrauterine growth restriction

E   There is reduced viscosity of secretions in the respiratory tract and pancreas

13.

i)

ii)

A   True ❑   False ❑

B   True ❑   False ❑

C   True ❑   False ❑

D   True ❑   False ❑

E   True ❑   False ❑

iii)

A   True ❑   False ❑

B   True ❑   False ❑

C   True ❑   False ❑

D   True ❑   False ❑

E   True ❑   False ❑

14.

A   True ❑   False ❑

B   True ❑   False ❑

C   True ❑   False ❑

D   True ❑   False ❑

E   True ❑   False ❑

1. i)   **C.** Exudative tonsillitis
      In diphtheria a thick grey pharyngeal membrane is characteristic.
      In acute epiglottitis the tonsils look normal. Examination of the throat is contraindicated as it may precipitate airway obstruction.
      Herpes simplex infection usually affects the lips, gums and tongue.
      Chicken pox is vesicular and mainly affects the hard palate.
   ii) Group A beta haemolytic streptococcus
      Epstein–Barr virus.

2. i)   Viral croup (laryngotracheobronchitis).
   ii) Inhalation of warm humidified air. Widely used but of unproven efficacy.
      Corticosteroids – nebulised or systemic.
      Nebulised adrenaline – provides transient relief in severe croup.
      Oxygen – hypoxaemia indicates severe airways obstruction.
      Tracheal intubation – this is required in 2–3% of children admitted to hospital.

3. **D.** This shows the characteristic grossly enlarged 'cherry red' epiglottis in acute epiglottitis.

4. i)   Subconjunctival haemorrhage.
   ii) Severe coughing or vomiting, e.g. pertussis
      Trauma (including non-accidental injury)
      Thrombocytopenia or platelet function disorder.

5. **D.** This allows the pathogen (*Bordetella pertussis*) to be identified.
   A marked lymphocytosis is characteristic but not diagnostic of pertussis.
   Immunofluorescence of a nasopharyngeal aspirate is used to identify respiratory syncitial virus, but is not helpful in the diagnosis of pertussis.
   These chest X-ray changes can occur in whooping cough but are not diagnostic.

6. i)   Bronchiolitis.
   ii) Marked respiratory distress (tachypnoea and severe intercostal recession)
      Poor feeding
      Past history of prematurity.

   iii) Humidified oxygen.

7. i)   **A** *False.* The percussion note would be stony dull.
      B *True.* He has focal chest signs.
      C *False.*
      D *False.* He has already failed to respond to two courses of antibiotics.
      E *False.*
   ii) Inhalation of a foreign body at his birthday party, e.g. peanut.

8.

Case history	A	B	C	D	Most likely diagnosis
1				✓	Cystic fibrosis. There are large volume lungs with extensive reticulonodular shadowing and peribronchial thickening with hilar lymphadenopathy.
2	✓				Inhaled tooth. The tooth is visible in the right main bronchus.
3		✓			Pneumonia. There is loss of contour of the left heart border and of the left hemidiaphragm
4			✓		Heart failure. There is cardiomegaly and increased pulmonary vascular markings. This is most often from a VSD.

9. A *True.*
    B. *False.* There is also inflammation of the bronchial mucosa.
    C *True.*
    D *True.*
    E *False.* Asthma is episodic, so peak flow may be normal when tested. Also, a peak flow may fall within the normal range for the population but be suboptimal for a particular child.

10. C.
    Metered dose inhaler (MDI) alone requires too much co-ordination for this age group.
    Dry powder inhaler is appropriate only for school-age children (over about six years).
    Oral treatment with tablets or syrup is ineffective.

11. i) A *False.* Her attack is severe as she is unable to complete a sentence.
        B *False.* The absence of wheeze in these circumstances implies that little air is moving in and out of the chest and would indicate a severe exacerbation.
        C *False.* Sitting assists lung mechanics and enables her to use her accessory muscles.
        D *True.*
        E *False.* The priority is to treat her asthma. If a chest X-ray is indicated, it must be taken in the A and E department.
    ii) A *True.*
        B *True.*
        C *True.*
        D *False.* She should be given humidified 100% oxygen by face mask.
        E *False.* Nebulised salbutamol can be administered continuously if necessary.

12. A *False.* Clubbing suggests suppurative lung disease or congenital heart disease.
    B *False.* This suggests suppurative lung disease.
    C *True.*
    D *False.* Static weight only occurs in asthma when it is very severe and uncontrolled.
    E *True.*

13. i) Poor weight gain since birth
        History of being 'always chesty'
        Irish descent. The gene frequency is particularly high in Ireland.
    ii) A *False.*
        B *False.*
        C *True.*
        D *False.*
        E *True.*
    iii) A *False.* He requires a high energy diet.
         B *True.*
         C *False.* Fat soluble vitamin supplements are required.
         D *True.*
         E *True.*

14. A *True.*
    B *True.* This is caused by an abnormality in the cystic fibrosis transmembrane regulator (CFTR).
    C *False.* The diagnosis is made on the sweat test although gene analysis is being increasingly used.
    D *False.* Failure to thrive occurs postnatally.
    E *False.* The viscosity of the secretions is markedly increased.

15 Cardiac disorders

1. *Regarding the foramen ovale:*
   i) What two factors cause it to close?
   ii) In what circumstances is it necessary to maintain the patency of the foramen ovale?

2. *When might it be desirable to keep the ductus arteriosus patent using drug therapy?*

3. *A systolic murmur is heard incidentally during an outpatient appointment. Which of the following features suggest that it requires further investigation:*
   A   A thrill
   B   Sinus arrhythmia on ECG
   C   Disappearance on lying flat
   D   An additional soft diastolic murmur
   E   Shortness of breath on exercise

4. *In a newborn infant, what bedside test allows the differentiation of cardiac from respiratory cyanosis?*

5. *Sarah was born at term by spontaneous vaginal delivery and went home on the second day of life following a normal neonatal discharge examination. On the 4th day her mother found her looking pale and was unable to wake her. She was rushed to the Accident and Emergency department. Her breathing was noted to be very shallow, her skin was cool and mottled and she was unresponsive to pain.*
   i) How would you describe her clinical state?
   ii) List the two most likely diagnoses to account for her sudden collapse:

   She is resuscitated, placed on a ventilator, given intravenous fluids and broad spectrum antibiotics. On re-examination, the only palpable pulse is the right brachial.

   iii) What is the most likely diagnosis?
   iv) What simple clinical measurement might help to confirm the diagnosis?

Answer column:

1 i)

   ii)

2.

3.
A True ❏   False ❏
B True ❏   False ❏
C True ❏   False ❏
D True ❏   False ❏
E True ❏   False ❏

4.

5. i)

    ii)

    iii)

    iv)

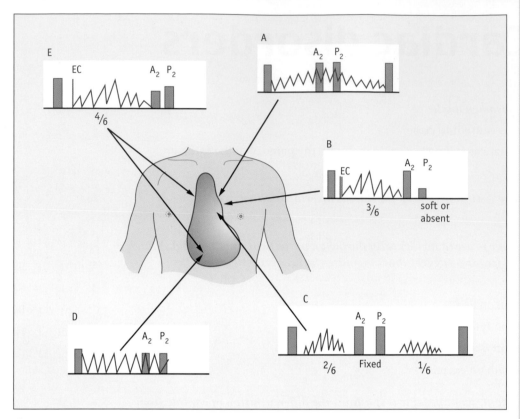

Fig. 15.1

6. *Complete the following table to indicate which murmur (Fig. 15.1) corresponds with the lesions listed.*

6.

	A	B	C	D	E
Atrial septal defect (ASD)					
Ventricular septal defect (VSD)					
Patent ductus arteriosus (PDA)					
Pulmonary valve stenosis					
Aortic valve stenosis					

7. *Ben, aged two months, is admitted with tachypnoea following an upper respiratory tract infection. On examination there is a thrill, a loud (Grade 4/6) pansystolic murmur at the left sternal edge and the liver is palpable 4 cm below the costal margin. The chest X-ray is shown (Fig. 15.2).*

i) What is the most likely cause of his clinical condition?

ii) What is the most likely underlying diagnosis?

iii) Why did he not develop symptoms immediately after birth?

iv) What is his likely long-term prognosis?

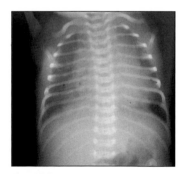

Fig. 15.2

7. i)

    ii)

    iii)

    iv)

8. *Which of the following statements about ventricular septal defects are true or false:*

A The louder the murmur, the larger the defect

B A loud second heart sound indicates pulmonary hypertension

C A large left to right shunt may result in pulmonary hypertension

D The Eisenmenger syndrome, with cyanosis from intracardiac right to left shunting, usually presents in infancy

E Antibiotic prophylaxis should be given to prevent bacterial endocarditis

8.

A True ❑ False ❑

B True ❑ False ❑

C True ❑ False ❑

D True ❑ False ❑

E True ❑ False ❑

9. *Which of the following statements about congenital heart disease are true or false:*

A In atrial septal defects (ASD), recurrent wheeze is a recognised presentation in childhood

B In asymptomatic children, closure of atrial septal defects is usually performed to prevent bacterial endocarditis in later life

C Older children with patent ductus arteriosus (PDA) may be treated with indomethacin (a prostaglandin synthetase inhibitor)

D In aortic valve stenosis, syncope is a recognised presentation

E In coarctation of the aorta, 'rib notching' may be observed in infancy

9.

A True ❑ False ❑

B True ❑ False ❑

C True ❑ False ❑

D True ❑ False ❑

E True ❑ False ❑

10. *Jason, aged eight months, is known to have Tetralogy of Fallot. His mother notices that he suddenly becomes dusky while waiting in the outpatient department.*

i) What is the pathophysiological basis of this episode?

ii) He is placed in the 'knee-chest position' but this does not help. Select from the list below the most appropriate further management:

   A Prostaglandin infusion

   B Immersion of the face in cold water

   C Intravenous morphine

   D Intravenous antibiotics

   E DC shock

10. i)

   ii) A B C D E

11. *David, aged six weeks, presents with sweating and poor feeding for 12 hours. He was born at term by spontaneous vaginal delivery, and has been a thriving, healthy baby. On examination in the Accident and Emergency department it is noted that he has cool peripheries and a fast, thready pulse. An ECG is performed and is shown in Fig. 15.3.*

i) What is the rhythm?

ii) What initial manoeuvre should be performed to attempt to restore sinus rhythm?

iii) What is the drug treatment of first choice?

11. i)

   ii)

   iii)

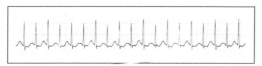

Fig. 15.3

12. *Which of the following statements about rheumatic fever are true or false:*

A It is an abnormal immune response to a previous pneumococcal infection

B It mainly affects school-age children of 5–15 years of age

C The arthritis characteristically affects the sacroiliac joint

D Erythema marginatum and subcutaneous nodules are major manifestations for the diagnosis

E The most frequent long-term damage is aortic stenosis

13. *Which of the following are manifestations of bacterial endocarditis:*

A Microscopic haematuria

B Sydenham's chorea

C Small necrotic skin lesions

D Splenomegaly

E Acute hemiplegia

14. *What two pieces of advice should be given to minimise the risk of bacterial endocarditis in children who have congenital heart disease?*

12.

A True ❑ False ❑

B True ❑ False ❑

C True ❑ False ❑

D True ❑ False ❑

E True ❑ False ❑

13.

A True ❑ False ❑

B True ❑ False ❑

C True ❑ False ❑

D True ❑ False ❑

E True ❑ False ❑

14.

1. i) Increased left atrial pressure. When the lungs fill with air, blood flow through the lungs via the pulmonary veins into the left atrium increases markedly.
        Reduced right atrial pressure. The expansion of the lungs reduces pulmonary artery resistance causing a fall in pressure in the right side of the heart.
    ii) To allow mixing between the pulmonary and systemic circulation in transposition of the great arteries.

2. If either the pulmonary blood flow, e.g. in pulmonary atresia, or the systemic blood flow, for example in severe coarctation of the aorta, is insufficient.
    Maintaining the patency of the ductus arteriosus allows blood to bypass the lesion.

3. A *True.*
    B *False.* This is a variation in heart rate with respiration and is a normal finding in children.
    C *False.* This is characteristic of a venous hum which is innocent.
    D *True.* A diastolic murmur must always be investigated.
    E *True.* Cardiac symptoms in association with a murmur always warrants further investigation.

4. The hyperoxia test. The infant is placed in 100% oxygen for a minimum of 10 minutes. The cyanosis of cardiac origin cannot be overcome by increasing the inspired oxygen concentration, unlike in respiratory disease.

5. i) Shock.
    ii) i) Septicaemia/meningitis
         ii) Congenital heart disease
         iii) Inborn error of metabolism
    iii) Severe coarctation of the aorta or interrupted aortic arch. As the ductus arteriosus closes, perfusion of the left arm and lower body is compromised.
    iv) The lower limb blood pressure will be lower than in the right arm.

6.

	A	B	C	D	E
Atrial septal defect (ASD)			✓		
Ventricular septal defect (VSD)				✓	
Patent ductus arteriosus (PDA)	✓				
Pulmonary valve stenosis		✓			
Aortic valve stenosis					✓

7. i) Heart failure, probably precipitated by an upper respiratory tract infection. The chest X-ray shows an enlarged heart.
    ii) Ventricular septal defect (VSD).
    iii) At birth, the pressure difference between the two ventricles is small and little blood will flow across the VSD. With the normal fall in pulmonary vascular resistance in the first few weeks, shunting of blood will increase progressively and heart failure may develop.
    v)   Good. The VSD will probably close spontaneously. Follow-up is required.

8. A *False.* Loud pansystolic murmurs are from small defects because of turbulent blood flow.
    B *True.* This is important to detect in infancy.
    C *True.*
    D *False.* It usually presents in the second decade, but should be avoidable.
    E *True.*

9.   **A**   *True.*
   B   *False.* It is performed to prevent right heart failure and arrhythmias in later life. The risk of bacterial endocarditis in ASD is very low as it is a low pressure lesion.
   C   *False.* Indomethacin is used in preterm infants to assist physiological closure; in older children there is a defect in the muscle of the duct and surgical closure is required.
   D   *True.*
   E   *False.* This is only seen in older children when large collateral arteries have developed.

10.   i)   This is a hypercyanotic spell due to spasm of the right ventricular outflow tract. There is a paroxysmal decrease in pulmonary artery blood flow with increased right to left shunting across the VSD.
   ii)   **C.** This relaxes the right ventricular outflow tract and will also calm him down.

11.   i)   Supraventricular tachycardia (SVT).
   ii)   Vagal stimulation, e.g. a bag of icy water can be placed on the face.
   iii)   Adenosine given as a rapid intravenous bolus.

12.   **A**   *False.* It follows a Group A β-haemolytic streptococcal infection rather than a pneumococcal infection.
   B   *True.*
   C   *False.* The arthritis mainly affects the ankles, knees and wrists.
   D   *True.*
   E   *False.* The commonest lesion is mitral stenosis, although any valve can be affected.

13.   **A**   *True.*
   B   *False.* It is a feature of rheumatic fever.
   C   *True.*
   D   *True.*
   E   *True.* From cerebral infarction.

14.   Good dental hygiene.
   Antibiotic prophylaxis for dental treatment and surgery which is likely to be associated with bacteraemia, i.e. oropharyngeal, gastrointestinal and genitourinary procedures or surgery.

16 Kidney and urinary tract

1. *Which of the following statements about renal physiology are true or false:*

   A The glomerular filtration rate during the first week of life is less than during adult life

   B The glomerular filtration rate cannot be measured in young children

   C The normal plasma creatinine is higher in infants than in adults

   D A plasma urea and creatinine in the normal range indicates normal renal function

   E In renal tubular acidosis, there is a metabolic acidosis and alkaline urine

1.

A True ☐   False ☐

B True ☐   False ☐

C True ☐   False ☐

D True ☐   False ☐

E True ☐   False ☐

2. *Which of the following are clinical features of urinary tract infections in an infant or a young child:*

   A Febrile convulsion

   B Petechiae

   C Vomiting

   D Abdominal pain

   E Recurrence of enuresis

2.

A True ☐   False ☐

B True ☐   False ☐

C True ☐   False ☐

D True ☐   False ☐

E True ☐   False ☐

3. *Lucie, aged one year, presents with a three-day history of fever. A bag urine is sent for analysis. Complete the table below by selecting the most likely interpretation of each urine examination result. More than one interpretation may apply.*

	Urine results				Interpretation of urine results			
	WBC mm³	RBC	Organisms/ Red cell casts	Culture	Perineal contamination	Urinary tract infection	Vulvo- vaginitis	Glomerulo- nephritis
A	100	–	–	–				
B	> 200	+++	–	>10⁵ coliforms				
C	< 50	–		Mixed coliforms				
D	50–100	+++	Red cell casts	–				
E	> 200	–	Organisms	>10⁵ coliforms				

4. *George, aged two months, has been off his feeds for 24 hours and has developed a fever of 39°C. On examination he is crying and cannot be consoled. No other abnormalities are noted.*

   The following investigations are performed:
   Hb 10.8 g/dl, WBC 17×10^9/l, platelets 424×10^9/l
   Blood culture – result awaited
   Chest X-ray – normal
   Lumbar puncture. Opening pressure – normal. CSF microscopy negative, glucose and protein concentrations normal.

An intravenous infusion is established. After waiting an hour for a urine sample without success, intravenous antibiotics are started.

The next morning a clean catch urine sample is obtained. It has > 200WBC/mm³ but no red cells. Microscopy shows no organisms and culture is subsequently negative.

i) Has a urinary tract infection been proven?

ii) How should the urine sample have been obtained in this situation?

iii) It had to be assumed that he had a urinary tract infection. Which of the following investigations are indicated?

    A Ultrasound of the kidneys and urinary tract

    B Intravenous urogram

    C Functional isotope scan (e.g. DMSA scan)

    D Indirect cystography

    E Direct cystography (MCUG)

5. *This is the ultrasound of the bladder (Fig. 16.1) and a micturating cystourethrogram (MCUG) (Fig. 16.2) in a newborn infant who was noted to have bilateral hydronephrosis on antenatal ultrasound. What is the most likely diagnosis?*

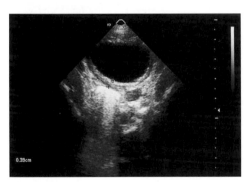

Fig. 16.1

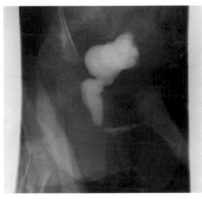

Fig. 16.2

6. *What abnormality is shown on this DMSA scan (Fig. 16.3) in a four-year-old girl who had a urinary tract infection three months' earlier?*

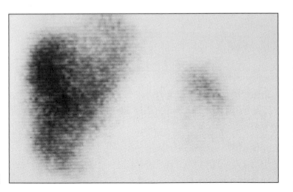

Fig. 16.3

4.

i) Yes ❏   No ❏

ii)

iii)

A True ❏   False ❏

B True ❏   False ❏

C True ❏   False ❏

D True ❏   False ❏

E True ❏   False ❏

5.

6.

7. *David, aged two years, has had a urinary tract infection and an abnormal DMSA scan. What is the major abnormality shown on this MCUG (Fig. 16.4)?*

7.

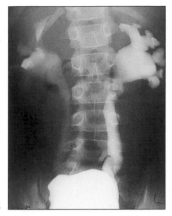

Fig. 16.4

8. *Which of the following statements about vesicoureteric reflux (VUR) are true or false:*

A There is usually an abnormality of the ureters where they enter the bladder

B The risk is increased if there are affected first-degree relatives

C The kidneys may be damaged when infected urine refluxes into them

D Renal scarring may result in hypertension

E The condition is usually permanent

8.

A True ❏   False ❏

B True ❏   False ❏

C True ❏   False ❏

D True ❏   False ❏

E True ❏   False ❏

9. *Three-year-old Paul was noted to have a swollen face on waking (Fig. 16.5). He had developed an upper respiratory tract infection a week earlier, from which he has recovered.*

List two conditions which may cause this appearance.

9.

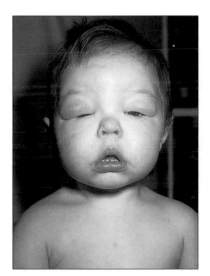

Fig. 16.5

10. *Joanne, aged four years, is newly diagnosed as having nephrotic syndrome. She has oedema of the eyelids and legs. Her blood pressure is 80/55 mmHg. Her plasma creatinine is normal for her age. The urine shows marked proteinuria but no haematuria.*

i) If a renal biopsy were performed, what would be the most likely finding on light microscopy?

ii) Joanne complains of abdominal pain.

List two complications of nephrotic syndrome associated with this symptom.

iii) She is started on corticosteroid therapy. What other therapy does she require while she remains hypoalbuminaemic?

10. i)

ii)

iii)

11. *Parviz, aged seven years, develops dark red urine. He had a sore throat two weeks ago. He has a temperature of 37.2°C, blood pressure 105/70. Examination is otherwise normal.*

    i)   What is the most likely diagnosis?

    ii) List two investigations to confirm it.

    iii) Name one acute complication.

    iv) What is the prognosis of this condition?

11. i)

    ii)

    iii)

    iv)

12. *This boy has haematuria (Fig. 16.6). What is the most likely diagnosis?*

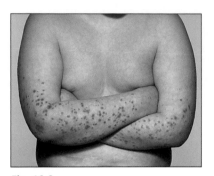

Fig. 16.6

12.

13. *Which of the following statements about Henoch–Schönlein purpura are true or false:*

    A It is a vasculitis

    B The rash characteristically involves the buttocks and legs

    C Abdominal colic is a recognised feature

    D Microscopic haematuria usually resolves spontaneously

    E It is associated with a prolonged prothrombin time

13.

A True ❑ False ❑

B True ❑ False ❑

C True ❑ False ❑

D True ❑ False ❑

E True ❑ False ❑

14. *Zahra, aged four years, presents with a two-day history of bloody diarrhoea. Over the previous 12 hours she has become increasingly unwell and has passed little urine.*

    Full blood count –
    Hb 8 g/dl, WBC 14 × 10⁹/l, platelet count 70 × 10⁹/l
    Plasma creatinine 200 μmol/l (normal 20–80 μmol/l)

    i)   What is the most likely diagnosis?

    ii) Which pathogen is associated with this disorder?

14. i)

    ii)

15. *Which of the following statements about hypertension are true or false:*

    A The normal range of blood pressure in children is related to height

    B The optimal blood pressure cuff size is one that covers one-third of the length of the upper arm length

    C It is associated with vesicoureteric reflux

    D Retinopathy is a recognised feature in children

    E It is associated with coarctation of the aorta

15.

A True ❑ False ❑

B True ❑ False ❑

C True ❑ False ❑

D True ❑ False ❑

E True ❑ False ❑

1. A   *True.* It is only 15% of the normal adult value.
   B   *False.* It can be measured but has the disadvantage that it requires an injection followed by several timed blood samples.
   C   *False.* Although renal function is less than in adults, their creatinine is lower as they have less muscle bulk.
   D   *False.* The plasma urea and creatinine concentration only rise once renal function is less than half of its normal value.
   E   *True.*

2. A   *True.*
   B   *False.*
   C   *True.*
   D   *True.*
   E   *True.*

3.

	Urine results				Interpretation of urine results			
	WBC mm³	RBC	Organisms/ Red cell casts	Culture	Perineal contamination	Urinary tract infection	Vulvo- vaginitis	Glomerulo- nephritis
A	100	–	–	–	✓		✓	
B	> 200	+++	–	>10⁵ coliforms		✓		
C	< 50	–		Mixed coliforms	✓			
D	50–100	+++	Red cell casts	–				✓
E	> 200	–	Organisms	>10⁵ coliforms		✓		

4. i)   No. The urine culture is negative but was obtained after antibiotics were started.
   ii) Suprapubic aspiration or catheter sample prior to antibiotics.
   iii) A   *True.*
        B   *False.*
        C   *True.*
        D   *False.* It is not possible to perform indirect cystography at this age as continence is required.
        E   *True.*

5. Posterior urethral valve. The ultrasound shows a thickened bladder wall and dilated ureter. The MCUG shows dilatation of the proximal urethra.

6. Severe scarring of the right kidney and scars at the upper and lower poles of the left kidney.

7. Bilateral gross vesicoureteric reflux. There is also clubbing of the renal calyces on the left.

8. A   *True.*
   B   *True.*
   C   *True.*
   D   *True.*
   E   *False.* It usually resolves during childhood.

9. Nephrotic syndrome – the most likely diagnosis
   Acute glomerulonephritis
   Angioedema.

10. i)   It is likely to be normal as her most likely diagnosis is minimal change glomerulonephritis. An abnormality (podocyte fusion) is only apparent on electron microscopy.
    ii) Hypovolaemia
         Peritonitis
         Renal vein thrombosis.
    iii) Penicillin prophylaxis against pneumococcal infection.

11. i)   Post-streptococcal glomerulonephritis.
    ii) Urine microscopy – red cells and casts
         ASO titre and throat swab – for streptococcal infection
         Complement levels – C_3 is initially low.
    iii) Seizures – because of hypertension
         Heart failure – from volume overload
         Acute renal failure – rare.
    iv) Excellent.

12. Henoch–Schönlein purpura.

13. A *True.*
    B *True.*
    C *True.*
    D *True.*
    E *False.* Coagulation is normal. The rash is due to a vasculitis.

14. i)   Acute renal failure from haemolytic uraemic syndrome (HUS).
    ii) *E. Coli* (0157 H7) or, less often, Shigella.

15. A *True.*
    B *False.* The cuff should cover at least two-thirds of the upper arm.
    C *True.* This may be secondary to renal scarring.
    D *True.*
    E *True.*

17 Genitalia

1. *Which of these statements about undescended testes are true or false:*

A An undescended testis is a normal variant in an infant less than 32 weeks' gestation

B A retractile testis is likely to require an orchidopexy

C Undescended testes are best corrected before two years of age to optimise fertility

D Impalpable testes must be identified surgically as they are at increased risk of undergoing malignant change

E Ectopic testes do not produce testosterone in response to intramuscular human chorionic gonadotrophin (hCG)

2. *Garry, aged four months, is referred urgently to outpatients because of an intermittent swelling in both groins (Fig. 17.1).*

i) What is the diagnosis?

ii) What is the management?

iii) If this lesion became red and painful, what complication would you suspect?

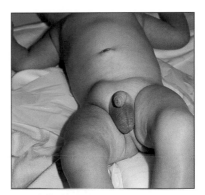

Fig. 17.1

3. *What is the anatomical difference between an inguinal hernia in an infant and in an adult?*

4. *This lesion (Fig. 17.2a) was identified on routine neonatal examination. Fig. 17.2b shows it on transillumination.*

   What is the diagnosis?

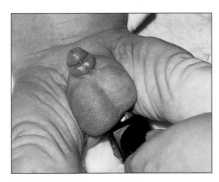

Fig. 17.2a

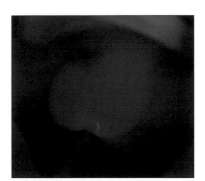

Fig. 17.2b

1.

A True ☐ False ☐

B True ☐ False ☐

C True ☐ False ☐

D True ☐ False ☐

E True ☐ False ☐

2. i)

ii)

iii)

3. Infant

Adult

4.

5. *Jean-Paul, aged 13 years, has developed an acutely painful red scrotum.*

i) What is the most important diagnosis to consider?

ii) List two other diagnoses you would consider.

iii) How would you manage this child?

6. *Fig. 17.3*

i) What is this condition (Fig. 17.3)?

ii) What procedure is contraindicated?

5. i)

ii)

iii)

6. i)

ii)

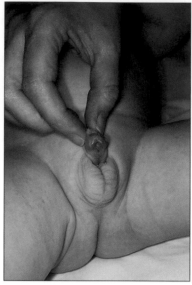

Fig. 17.3

7. *Which of these statements about conditions affecting the genitalia are true or false:*

A Vulvovaginitis is a recognised cause of dysuria

B A vaginal discharge in a young child is indicative of sexual abuse

C Female infants with bilateral inguinal hernias require chromosomal analysis

D Inguinal hernias are commoner in preterm than term infants

E Acute balanitis is an indication for circumcision

7.

A True ❑ False ❑

B True ❑ False ❑

C True ❑ False ❑

D True ❑ False ❑

E True ❑ False ❑

1. **A** *True.*
    B *False.* Treatment is not required if the testis can be brought into the base of the scrotum without tension.
    C *True.*
    D *True.*
    E *False.* This may be used as a test to confirm the presence of testicular tissue irrespective of its site.

2. i)   Bilateral inguinal hernia.
    ii) Surgical repair. It should be performed promptly, i.e. on the next routine surgical list.
    iii) Strangulation of the bowel or testis.

3. Infant – it is caused by a patent processus vaginalis and always indirect.
    Adult – due to a muscular defect of the inguinal canal and may be direct or indirect.

4. Bilateral hydroceles.

5. i)   Torsion of the testis.
    ii) Torsion of the appendage of the testis
         Epididymitis
         Strangulated inguinal hernia.
    iii) Urgent surgical exploration is required. If immediately available the diagnosis of torsion of testis can be confirmed using Doppler ultrasound.

6. i)   Hypospadias with chordee.
    ii) Circumcision.

7. **A** *True.*
    B *False.* Vaginal discharge is relatively common. Although it may result from sexual abuse, idiopathic vulvovaginitis and urethritis are much more common.
    C *True.* Inguinal hernias are uncommon in females, and when bilateral may be a feature of intersex.
    D *True.*
    E *False.* Balanitis is usually an isolated event and so circumcision is indicated only if it occurs recurrently.

18 Liver disorders

1. **Which of the following are signs of chronic liver disease in children:**

A Bruising

B Clubbing

C Splenomegaly

D Erythema multiforme

E Encephalopathy

2. *Reece, aged four weeks, is taken to his general practitioner because he is jaundiced. He was born at term and is formula-fed. His mother reports that he has always looked yellow but is now feeding less well.*

   Which of the following should be considered in the differential diagnosis:

i) A Breast-milk jaundice

    B Urinary tract infection

    C Hypothyroidism

    D Sickle cell disease

    E Biliary atresia

ii) What further history would suggest that the jaundice is obstructive?

iii) What blood test would you perform to confirm that the jaundice is obstructive?

iv) Obstructive jaundice is confirmed. What diagnosis needs to be rapidly excluded?

3. *Raj, a 14-year-old boy, is noted to be jaundiced. He has recently returned from India where he was visiting relatives in a rural village.*

i) Select the two viruses most likely to have caused his jaundice:

    A Hepatitis A

    B Hepatitis B

    C Hepatitis C

    D Hepatitis D

    E Hepatitis E

ii) List two non-infectious alternative diagnoses:

4. **Which of the following statements about hepatitis are true or false:**

A The absence of jaundice excludes the diagnosis of hepatitis A.

B Chronic liver disease characteristically follows hepatitis A.

C Infants who acquire hepatitis B by vertical transmission characteristically develop acute hepatitis in the first year of life.

D Infants born to HBsAg positive mothers should receive a course of hepatitis B vaccination starting shortly after birth.

E Infants with hepatitis C are at increased risk of chronic liver disease.

1.

A True ☐ False ☐

B True ☐ False ☐

C True ☐ False ☐

D True ☐ False ☐

E True ☐ False ☐

2. i)

A True ☐ False ☐

B True ☐ False ☐

C True ☐ False ☐

D True ☐ False ☐

E True ☐ False ☐

ii)

iii)

iv)

3. i) A B C D E

   ii)

4.

A True ☐ False ☐

B True ☐ False ☐

C True ☐ False ☐

D True ☐ False ☐

E True ☐ False ☐

5. *Ben, aged nine months, has had a Kasai procedure (hepatoportoenterostomy) for biliary atresia. Subsequently he develops cirrhosis, is failing to thrive and is on the waiting list for a liver transplant.*

i) Give two reasons for Ben's failure to thrive.

ii) Give two interventions which may improve his growth:

6. *Stacey, aged 14 years, has taken 30–40 paracetamol tablets, washed down with a quantity of 'Alco-pop'.*

i) What antidote would you give her?

ii) Although she is initially asymptomatic, at around 36 hours after the ingestion, she develops right upper quadrant abdominal pain. Investigations reveal a rise in her bilirubin and liver transaminases. Which of these statements about the management of her acute liver failure are true or false:

A   Albumin is the best indicator of her liver function.

B   Hypoglycaemia is a recognised complication.

C   Confusion requires prompt psychiatric evaluation.

D   Prothrombin time is a useful prognostic marker.

E   She should be given vitamin K.

7. *Summer, aged four months, is seen in the Accident and Emergency department with a two-day history of nasal discharge and four hours of breathlessness. Examination findings are shown in Fig. 18.1.*

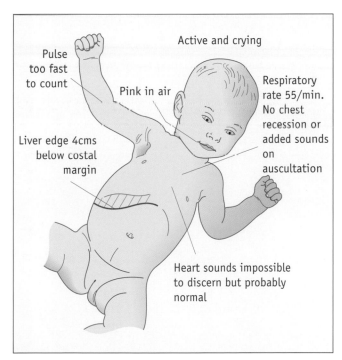

Active and crying

Pulse too fast to count

Pink in air

Respiratory rate 55/min. No chest recession or added sounds on auscultation

Liver edge 4cms below costal margin

Heart sounds impossible to discern but probably normal

Fig. 18.1

What is the most likely cause of her hepatomegaly?

---

5. i)

ii)

6.
i)

ii)

A   True ❑   False ❑

B   True ❑   False ❑

C   True ❑   False ❑

D   True ❑   False ❑

E   True ❑   False ❑

7.

8. *Fig. 18.2*

i) What is this sign?

ii) What is the underlying diagnosis?

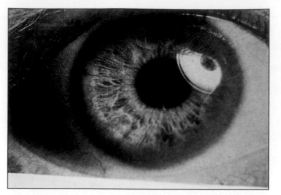

Fig. 18.2

8. i)

ii)

1. **A** *True.*
   B *True.*
   C *True.*
   D *False.*
   E *True.*

2. i) **A** *False.* He is bottle-fed!
      B *True.*
      C *True.*
      D *False.* Sickle cell disease does not cause symptoms or signs until fetal haemoglobin is replaced by adult haemoglobin at several months of age.
      E *True.*
   ii) Pale stools and dark urine.
   iii) Measure the conjugated bilirubin. Jaundice is obstructive if more than 20% of the total bilirubin is conjugated.
   iv) Biliary atresia. Early surgery improves prognosis.

3. i) A and E. Hepatitis A and E are spread by the faecal/oral route where sanitation is poor. Hepatitis B, C and D are spread by contaminated body fluids, e.g. blood.
   ii) Haemolytic anaemia e.g. G6PD deficiency
      Drug reaction
      Autoimmune hepatitis
      Gall stones
      Rare metabolic conditions e.g. Wilson's disease.

4. **A** *False.* 30%–50% of children with hepatitis A do not develop jaundice.
   B *False.* Hepatitis A does not cause chronic liver disease.
   C *False.* Infants who acquire the hepatitis B virus by vertical transmission are usually asymptomatic carriers.
   D *True.*
   E *True.*

5. i) Anorexia.
      Fat malabsorption and deficiencies in fat soluble vitamins (A, D, E and K) due to biliary tract obstruction.
      Increased energy requirement.
   ii) Calorie supplementation with a diet rich in protein and carbohydrate.
      Fat soluble vitamin supplementation.
      Nasogastric feeding.

6. i) Intravenous N-acetylcysteine.
   ii) **A** *False.* Albumin has a long half-life, therefore the serum level does not fall acutely.
      B *True.*
      C *False.* Her confusion is likely to be the result of the encephalopathy of acute liver failure.
      D *True.* Prothrombin time is the most helpful acute measure of liver function.
      E *True.*

7. Cardiac failure secondary to supraventricular tachycardia.

8. i) Kayser–Fleischer ring.
   ii) Wilson's disease.

19 Malignant disease

1. *Which of the following statements about malignant disease are true or false:*

A Leukaemia is the commonest malignancy in childhood

B More children die from malignant disease than accidents

C Neutropenic children who develop a fever should be treated promptly with oral antibiotics

D Infertility is a recognised side effect of chemotherapy using an alkylating agent

E After 15 years' survival from acute lymphoblastic leukaemia, the risk of developing a tumour is the same as the general population

2. *Which one of the following is the biochemical marker of neuroblastoma:*

A Urinary catecholamines

B Serum β-HCG (human chorionic gonadotrophin)

C Plasma LDH (lactate dehydrogenase)

D Plasma ammonia

E Serum α-fetoprotein

3. *Which of the following statements about leukaemia and lymphoma in children are true or false:*

A Acute myeloid leukaemia is the commonest form of leukaemia

B In leukaemia a low haemoglobin and platelet count are characteristically present at diagnosis

C Allopurinol is given before induction therapy is started

D Cotrimoxazole is given during continuing therapy

E Hodgkin's disease characteristically presents in pre-school children

4. *Frank, aged three, has had several respiratory infections during the last four months. He has become lethargic and developed a widespread petechial rash. His mother is worried that he may have leukaemia.*

i) List three signs on clinical examination which would support his mother's suspicion.

A blood film shows Hb 5.3 g/l, WBC 3.6 × 10⁹/l, platelets 22 × 10⁹/l.

ii) How would you describe these haematological findings?

iii) Select one further investigation required to confirm the diagnosis:

   A Mantoux test

   B Bone marrow examination

   C Urinary catecholamines

   D EBV titre

   E Chest X-ray

1.

A True ☐   False ☐

B True ☐   False ☐

C True ☐   False ☐

D True ☐   False ☐

E True ☐   False ☐

2. A   B   C   D   E

3.

A True ☐   False ☐

B True ☐   False ☐

C True ☐   False ☐

D True ☐   False ☐

E True ☐   False ☐

4.

i)

ii)

iii) A   B   C   D   E

5. *List the four key phases of treatment of acute lymphoblastic leukaemia.*

6. *Molly, aged four years, is on continuing (maintenance) therapy for acute lymphoblastic leukaemia. Her younger brother developed the rash shown in Fig. 19.1.*

i) What is this rash?

   Molly is well in herself but two weeks later also develops a rash. She has a fever of 37.9°C, respiratory rate of 40/minute, heart rate 136/minute and has laboured breathing. An oxygen saturation in air is 90%.

ii) What is the most likely cause of her illness?

iii) List two important therapies for her condition.

iv) How might her illness have been prevented?

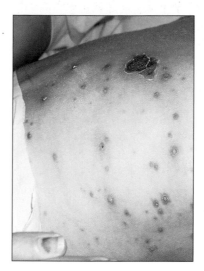

Fig. 19.1

7. *Jack, aged eight years, presents to his general practitioner with a two-week history of daily, severe headaches which have woken him at night. He has also become unsteady. Examination of his eyes is shown in Fig. 19.2. His cranial CT scan is shown in Fig. 9.3.*

i) Describe the abnormal sign demonstrated in the diagram (Fig. 9.2).

ii) What is the most likely diagnosis?

iii) What is the significance of the eye signs?

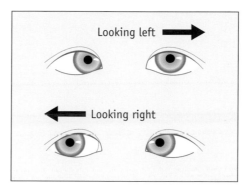

Fig. 19.2

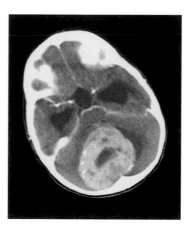

Fig. 19.3

5.

6. i)

ii)

iii)

iv)

7. i)

ii)

iii)

8. *Which of the following are characteristic presenting features of brain tumours?*

A Change in behaviour

B Visual field defect

C Headache accompanied by seeing flashing lights

D Ataxia

E Neck stiffness

8.

A True ❑   False ❑

B True ❑   False ❑

C True ❑   False ❑

D True ❑   False ❑

E True ❑   False ❑

9. *Complete the following table showing which features support a diagnosis of Wilms' tumour and which suggest neuroblastoma?*

9.

Presenting feature	Wilms' tumour	Neuroblastoma
Haematuria		
Abdominal mass extending beyond the midline		
Hepatomegaly		
Bone pain		
Spinal cord compression		

1. **A** *True.*
   B *False.* Many more children die from accidents than malignant disease.
   C *False.* Such children should always be assessed, cultures performed and given intravenous antibiotics.
   D *True.*
   E *False.* Long-term survivors are at increased risk of second tumours.

2. **A**. Urinary catecholamines.

3. **A** *False.* Acute lymphoblastic leukaemia accounts for 80% of leukaemia in children.
   B *True.*
   C *True.* This protects the kidneys from a rapid rise in uric acid from lysis of malignant cells.
   D *True.* This is to prevent *Pneumocystis carinii* pneumonia.
   E *False.* The commonest age of presentation is in teenagers and young adults.

4. i) Pallor from anaemia
   Marked lymphadenopathy
   Hepatosplenomegaly
   Bruising in addition to the petechiae
   Evidence of infection.
   ii) Pancytopenia.
   iii) **B**.

5. Remission induction
   Intensification
   CNS protection
   Continuing treatment.

6. i) Chicken pox.
   ii) Chicken pox pneumonitis. This is a serious condition in immunocompromised patients
   iii) Humidified oxygen
   Intravenous aciclovir.
   iv) At diagnosis, her chicken pox (and measles) antibody levels would have been checked. If she had been known to be susceptible, she should have been given zoster immune globulin following her contact with chicken pox.

7. i) Left VIth nerve palsy.
   ii) Brain tumour in the posterior fossa. The CT shows a large mass in the posterior fossa and dilated ventricles from hydrocephalus.
   iii) False localising sign from raised intracranial pressure.

8. **A** *True.*
   B *True.* The classical deficit is bitemporal hemianopia from a pituitary tumour, e.g. craniopharyngioma.
   C *False.* This is typical of migraine.
   D *True.* This is characteristic of a posterior fossa tumour, e.g. medulloblastoma.
   E *False.*

9.

Presenting feature	Wilms' tumour	Neuroblastoma
Haematuria	✓	
Abdominal mass extending beyond the midline		✓
Hepatomegaly		✓
Bone pain		✓
Spinal cord compression		✓

20 Haematology

1. *Which of the following statements about haemoglobin are true or false*

   A Fetal haemoglobin (HbF) has a lower oxygen affinity than adult haemoglobin

   B HbF is replaced by HbA during the first year of life

   C The red cell life span is shorter in the newborn period than in adults

   D Beyond infancy, a raised HbF is consistent with the diagnosis of a haemoglobinopathy

   E The haemoglobin concentration at birth is higher in growth restricted than in normal infants

1.

A True ☐ False ☐

B True ☐ False ☐

C True ☐ False ☐

D True ☐ False ☐

E True ☐ False ☐

2. *Joseph, a two-year old Afro-Caribbean, is admitted to hospital for the elective repair of an inguinal hernia. He has no other medical problems. Preoperative assessment reveals:*

   Hb 8.6 g/dl
   MCV 68 fl (normal 75–87 fl)
   MCHC 22 g/dl (normal 32–35 g/dl)
   WBC $11.2 \times 10^9/l$
   Platelets $262 \times 10^9/l$
   Hb electrophoresis – HbA 98%, HbA_2 2%

   This is his blood film (Fig. 20.1).

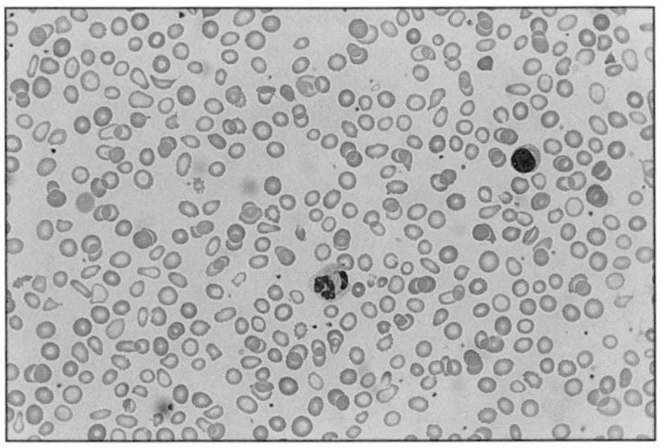

   i) What is the most likely cause of his anaemia?

   ii) What history is required to determine the underlying cause?

   iii) What further investigation would confirm your diagnosis?

Fig. 20.1

2. i)

    ii)

    iii)

3. *Which of the following statements about haemoglobinopathies are true or false:*

   A Fetal haemoglobin consists of two alpha and two gamma globin chains

   B In thalassaemia the structure of the globin chain is abnormal

   C In β-thalassaemia major the HbA_2 concentration is reduced

   D In β-thalassaemia the clinical severity depends on the amount of HbA and HbF present

   E In homozygous sickle cell disease (HbSS) there is HbS and HbF but no HbA

3.

A True ☐ False ☐

B True ☐ False ☐

C True ☐ False ☐

D True ☐ False ☐

E True ☐ False ☐

4. *Which of the following statements about haemolytic anaemias are true or false:*

   A Conjugated bilirubin is present in the urine

   B G6PD deficiency predisposes to oxidative damage to red blood cells

   C In G6PD deficiency only males are affected

   D Hereditary spherocytosis is autosomal dominant

   E In spherocytosis red blood cells have increased osmotic fragility

4.

A True ☐ False ☐

B True ☐ False ☐

C True ☐ False ☐

D True ☐ False ☐

E True ☐ False ☐

5. *Leon, a four-year old Afro-Caribbean boy, suddenly becomes pale, jaundiced and develops dark urine. This is his first illness since birth. Haemolysis from G6PD deficiency is suspected.*

i) How would you confirm the diagnosis?

ii) Name a possible precipitant for this episode.

6. *Amber, aged nine months, appears to be in pain. The appearance of her left hand is shown (Fig. 20.2). What is the most likely cause?*

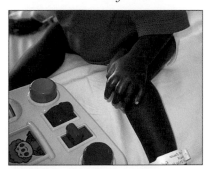

Fig. 20.2

7. *Complete the table to show which of the following are characteristic of homozygous sickle cell disease (HbSS) or β-thalassaemia major? Either, neither or both may be correct.*

	Sickle cell disease	β-thalassaemia major
Afro-Caribbean origin		
Greek Cypriot origin		
Autosomal recessive inheritance		
Anaemia in the neonatal period		
Splenic infarction		

8. *Ben, aged five years, with known homozygous sickle cell disease, presents with an increasingly painful right thigh and a temperature of 38°C. There is no history of trauma.*

i) List the two most likely causes of his leg pain.

ii) What are your two main treatment modalities and why?

9. *Shlomo, aged two weeks, continues to bleed following circumcision. Investigation reveals:*

Hb 11 g/dl, WBC 12 × 10^9/l, platelet count 322 × 10^9/l
PT 16 sec (control 15 sec)
APTT > 120 sec (control 27 sec)

Select the most likely diagnosis from the list below:

A Immune thrombocytopenic purpura (ITP)

B Haemophilia A

C Vitamin K deficiency

D Von Willebrand's disease

E Liver disease

5. i)

   ii)

6.

7.

8. i)

   ii)

9. A B C D E

10. *Charlie, aged five years, is troubled by recurrent nose bleeds, the last of which took 1½ hours to stop. Investigation shows:*

   Hb 8.6 g/dl, WBC 10.2 × 10⁹/l, platelets 350 × 10⁹/l
   PT 16 (control 15 sec)
   APTT 46 sec (control 28 sec)
   Fibrinogen 2.5 g/l (normal 2–4 g/l)
   Factor VIII:C low

   Select the most likely diagnosis from the list below:

   A   Immune thrombocytopenic purpura

   B   Haemophilia A

   C   Vitamin K deficiency

   D   Von Willebrand's disease

   E   Liver disease

11. *Ben's mother is concerned that he bruises easily (Fig. 20.3).*

   Which of the following conditions may cause this problem?

   A   Haemophilia A

   B   Acute liver failure

   C   Gentamicin therapy

   D   Acute lymphoblastic leukaemia (ALL)

   E   Henoch–Schönlein purpura (HSP)

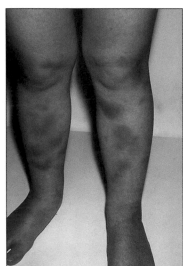

Fig. 20.3

11.

A   True ❑   False ❑
B   True ❑   False ❑
C   True ❑   False ❑
D   True ❑   False ❑
E   True ❑   False ❑

12. *Josephine, aged five years, develops purpura and bruises. She is otherwise well. There are no other abnormalities on examination. Investigation shows: Hb 11.8 g/dl, WBC 12.8 × 10⁹/l, platelets 28 × 10⁹/l. Immune thrombocytopenic purpura (ITP) is diagnosed.*

i)   Which of the following statements are true or false:

   A   If a bone marrow were performed, few megakaryocytes would be seen

   B   The most serious complication of her condition is intracranial haemorrhage

   C   A platelet infusion is indicated

   D   Her prognosis would be better if she were 15 years old

   E   Resolution of her condition within a few weeks is to be expected

ii) Which of the following are recognised forms of management of ITP:

   A   Bone marrow transplantation

   B   Corticosteroids

   C   Immunoglobulin

   D   Aspirin

   E   No active intervention

12.

i)

A   True ❑   False ❑
B   True ❑   False ❑
C   True ❑   False ❑
D   True ❑   False ❑
E   True ❑   False ❑

ii)

A   True ❑   False ❑
B   True ❑   False ❑
C   True ❑   False ❑
D   True ❑   False ❑
E   True ❑   False ❑

1. **A** *False*. HbF has a higher oxygen affinity to facilitate the transfer of oxygen from the maternal to the fetal circulation.
    B *True*.
    C *True*. This is one of the reasons why newborn infants often become jaundiced.
    D *True*.
    E *True*. This is to compensate for the lower oxygen tension in the growth-retarded fetus.

2. i)   Iron deficiency. The blood film shows a hypochromic, microcytic anaemia. This and the red cell indices are consistent with iron deficiency. β-thalassaemia trait is excluded by the normal Hb electrophoresis.
    ii) Dietary history to determine adequacy of iron intake.
    iii) Serum ferritin. This would be low.

3. **A** *True*.
    B *False*. In thalassaemia the **quantity** of globin chains produced is abnormal.
    C *False*. It is increased. There is a reduction in β-chain synthesis, so there is increased production of gamma and delta chains leading to higher levels of HbF and HbA_2 respectively.
    D *True*. The higher the levels of HbA and HbF, the milder the disease.
    E *True*.

4. **A** *False*. Urobilinogen is present.
    B *True*.
    C *False*. It is an X-linked disorder but homozygous females or heterozygotes with inactivation of the unaffected X chromosome (Lyonisation) may manifest the disease.
    D *True*.
    E *True*.

5. i)   Check a G6PD level following recovery of his haemolysis.
    ii) An acute infection
         Ingestion of certain drugs, e.g. primaquine
         Contact with naphthalene in moth balls
         Ingestion of fava beans in Mediterranean variants.

6. Dactylitis. This is likely to be from a vaso-occlusive crisis from homozygous sickle cell disease.

7.

	Sickle cell disease	β-thalassaemia major
Afro-Caribbean origin	✓	
Greek Cypriot origin		✓
Autosomal recessive inheritance	✓	✓
Anaemia in the neonatal period		
Splenic infarction	✓	

8. i)   Vaso-occlusive bone crisis
         Osteomyelitis.
    ii) Analgesia. Vaso-occlusive crises are often extremely painful and require opiates.
         Hydration. Dehydration may precipitate a crisis.
         Antibiotics if clinical evidence of osteomyelitis.

9. **B**.
    In ITP the platelet count would be low.
    In vitamin K deficiency and liver disease the PT would be prolonged.
    Severe Von Willebrand's disease could be a cause but is less likely than haemophilia A.

10. **D**. Von Willebrand's disease.

11. A *True.*
 B *True.*
 C *False.*
 D *True.*
 E *False.*

12. i) A *False.* The megakaryocytes are increased to try to compensate for the increased platelet destruction by the reticulo-endothelial system.
 B *True.* Fortunately it is very rare.
 C *False.* Platelets should only be given for acute haemorrhage as they are rapidly destroyed.
 D *False.*
 E *True.*

 ii) A *False.*
 B *True.*
 C *True.*
 D *False.*
 E *True.*

21 Emotions and behaviour

1. *Which of the following statements about a normal three-year-old child are true or false:*

    A   A consistent bedtime routine would be helpful if there was difficulty in settling him to sleep

    B   In the management of severe temper tantrums, a stimulant drug such as methylphenidate (Ritalin) might be indicated

    C   Blue breath-holding attacks can occur following frustration

    D   A bump on the head is a precipitating cause of white breath-holding attacks

    E   Biting a sibling is an indication for psychiatric evaluation

2. *Amy, aged nine years, is diagnosed as having leukaemia. Her parents ask for advice about what to tell her. Select which of the following statements are true or false:*

    A   She is too young to be told she has a serious illness

    B   She is too young to understand the concept of dying

    C   You would anticipate her asking her doctors lots of questions about her treatment

    D   Her 12-year-old brother should not be told the diagnosis

    E   The details of the treatment protocol should be fully explained to her

3. *Abdul-Aziz, aged 18 months, is brought to his general practitioner as his mother is concerned about his poor feeding. His personal child health record shows that he is following the 5th centile for length but the 0.4th centile for weight. Examination reveals an energetic, short, thin boy with no abnormalities. Which of the following statements are true or false:*

    A   His mother should be advised to improve his food intake by forcing food into his mouth

    B   Feeding via a nasogastric tube should be instituted

    C   A jejunal biopsy should be performed

    D   He should be punished if he fails to eat all the food on his plate

    E   He is starving himself deliberately to annoy his parents

4. *Jeremy, aged four years, is brought to his general practitioner because he wakes every night at about 10 p.m. with a shout. When his parents go to him he looks awake but confused. He goes back to sleep soon afterwards and next morning cannot recall any of these night-time events. Select the most likely explanation from the list below:*

    A   Nightmares

    B   Night terrors

    C   Complex partial seizures

    D   Motor tics

    E   Psychotic behaviour

Answer column

1.
A   True ☐   False ☐
B   True ☐   False ☐
C   True ☐   False ☐
D   True ☐   False ☐
E   True ☐   False ☐

2.
A   True ☐   False ☐
B   True ☐   False ☐
C   True ☐   False ☐
D   True ☐   False ☐
E   True ☐   False ☐

3.
A   True ☐   False ☐
B   True ☐   False ☐
C   True ☐   False ☐
D   True ☐   False ☐
E   True ☐   False ☐

4.   A   B   C   D   E

5. *The mother of Steven, aged three, is worried that he is not developing as rapidly as his older sister. He rarely says a word with meaning. At playschool he is always on his own and endlessly places a car in and out of a biscuit tin. If disturbed from doing this, he has a violent temper tantrum.*

i) Select the most likely diagnosis from the list below:

    A General learning disability

    B Hearing impairment

    C Obsessive compulsive disorder

    D Dyslexia

    E Autism

ii) Select one of the following investigations that needs to be performed:

    A Pituitary function tests

    B Hearing test

    C Visual acuity check

    D EEG

    E Skull X-ray

5. i) A B C D E
   ii) A B C D E

6. *Six-year-old Jennifer still wets the bed at night. She is about to go on a camping holiday. Complete the table below, selecting the form of therapy most likely to help her (i) be dry at the camp and (ii) provide long-term cure. Either, neither or both may be correct.*

6.

	Dry at camp	Long-term cure
A Phenobarbitone therapy		
B Sensor pad which causes an electric shock when wet		
C Punishment by withdrawing treats		
D Desmopressin therapy		
E Sensor pad which alarms when wet		

7. *Which of the following statements about defaecation are true or false:*

A Normal children should be out of nappies by their second birthday

B An anal fissure is a recognised cause of constipation

C Faecal retention can be readily cured with an enema alone

D Lactulose is a laxative which softens the stool and thereby aids voluntary defaecation

E An empty rectum suggests voluntary control over defaecation

7.

A True ❏ False ❏

B True ❏ False ❏

C True ❏ False ❏

D True ❏ False ❏

E True ❏ False ❏

8. *Which of the following statements about behavioural disorders in childhood are true or false:*

A Repeated frowning of the forehead and blinking of the eyes has a good prognosis

B Having difficulty with making friends is a feature of ADHD (Attention Deficit Hyperactivity Disorder)

C Recurrent pains in the legs are a recognised manifestation of anxiety

D Non-attendance at school because of recurrent headaches is called truancy

E Encopresis is the passage of stool in inappropriate places

8.

A True ❏ False ❏

B True ❏ False ❏

C True ❏ False ❏

D True ❏ False ❏

E True ❏ False ❏

9. *Which of the following statements about anorexia nervosa are true or false:*

A There is indifference to food

B Premature onset of puberty is a characteristic feature

C There is a preoccupation with weight

D It is associated with a past history of underachievement at school

E It is associated with amenorrhoea

10. *For the last three months Felicity, aged 13 years, has complained of difficulty in doing school work, increased tiredness on the slightest exercise, pain in her joints and headaches with tenderness over the top of her head. She has not attended school for the last month.*

10. i) **A B C D E**
   ii) **A B C D E**

i) On the basis of this history alone select the most likely diagnosis:

   A Tuberculosis

   B Brain tumour

   C Depression

   D Hypothyroidism

   E Chronic fatigue syndrome

ii) Examination and investigations reveal no abnormality. Select the most appropriate management:

   A Complete bed rest

   B Provide home tuition

   C Gradual rehabilitation

   D Intensive exercise

   E None of the above

11. *Sharon, aged 15 years, is admitted to hospital following an overdose of 10 paracetamol tablets. She makes an uneventful recovery. A more detailed history reveals that she has not been feeling herself for the past few months. She has had chest and stomach pains. Her mother relates that Sharon has been feeling down and uninterested in life. Her teachers are very concerned about the deterioration in her school performance.*

11. i) Yes ❏ No ❏
   ii) Yes ❏ No ❏
   iii) **A B C D E**

i) Is depression a possible diagnosis in a child of her age?

ii) Are most adolescents who take an overdose clinically depressed?

iii) Select the most appropriate management:

   A Reassure that this is a normal part of adolescence

   B Design a rehabilitation programme with her parents

   C Refer to a child psychiatrist

   D Perform a cranial CT scan

   E Request an EEG

12. *Sam, aged five years, is referred to outpatients by her general practitioner with a three-month history of abdominal pain. When asked where it hurts she points to her umbilicus. The pain occurs daily at varying times and might last up to 30 minutes. She has no bowel or urinary symptoms. Her past medical history is unremarkable. Examination including height and weight is normal.*

i) Name one further aspect of the history you would wish to elicit.

ii) Urine microscopy and culture are negative. Select the most appropriate further investigation from the following:

   A Jejunal biopsy

   B Plain abdominal X-ray

   C Serum amylase

   D Colonoscopy

   E None of the above

iii) Select the most appropriate management of this child:

   A Exclusion diet

   B Sulphasalazine treatment

   C Reassurance

   D Psychiatric assessment

   E Senna and lactulose therapy

12. i)

   ii) **A B C D E**

   iii) **A B C D E**

1. **A** *True.*
   B *False.* Behaviour modification should be used; methylphenidate (Ritalin) is used in attention deficit hyperactivity disorder (ADHD).
   C *True.*
   D *True.*
   E *False.* This is often encountered at this age.

2. **A** *False.*
   B *False.*
   C *False.* Children rarely ask questions in unfamiliar situations. They may question their parents later.
   D *False.* He needs to know why his sister needs so much parental attention and why hospital visits are causing so much family upset.
   E *False.* It is the concepts and not the details that are important to her and her family at this stage.

3. **A** *False.* This is likely to lead to him vomiting his food and may lead to meal refusal.
   B *False.* He does not require supplementary nutrition as he is not failing to thrive.
   C *False.* There is no suggestion of coeliac disease.
   D *False.* His mother is expecting him to eat more at mealtimes than he needs and she will not win these battles.
   E *False.* He is eating adequately to maintain normal growth.

4. **B.** This is typical of night terrors.
   Nightmares occur before waking and can usually be recalled.
   Complex partial seizures, motor tics and psychotic behaviour do not present in this way.

5. i) **E.**
   ii) **B.** All children with significant speech delay must have a hearing test.

6.

		Dry at camp	Long-term cure
A	Phenobarbitone therapy		
B	Sensor pad which causes an electric shock when wet		
C	Punishment by withdrawing treats		
D	Desmopressin therapy	✓	
E	Sensor pad which alarms when wet		✓

7. **A** *False.* By 3–4 years.
   B *True.* Due to pain.
   C *False.* Although this will empty the rectum the descending colon will remain distended and dysfunctional. Retraining is required.
   D *True.*
   E *True.*

8. **A** *True.* Tics of this nature have a good prognosis.
   B *True.*
   C *True.*
   D *False.* This is school refusal. Truancy is a conduct disorder.
   E *True.*

9. **A** *False.* There is a preoccupation with food.
   B *False.* Puberty is delayed.
   C *True.* This is associated with a disordered body image.
   D *False.* Affected children are characteristically compliant and hard-working at school.
   E *True.*

10. i) **E.** Chronic fatigue syndrome is the most likely diagnosis but other causes, particularly depression, should be considered.
    ii) **C.** Gradual rehabilitation is usually the most successful approach in chronic fatigue syndrome. This consists of a gradual increase in exercise, school work and normal daily living.

11. i) Yes. Depression, although uncommon, occurs even in children of primary school age.
    ii) No. But up to a third may be depressed.
    iii) **C.** She requires treatment of her depression.

12. i) Stress in the family or at school e.g. bullying.
    ii) **E.** There is no clinical evidence of an organic cause.
    iii) **C.**

22 Skin

1. *Which of the following statements about the skin in children is true or false:*

A The poorly keratinised skin of pre-term infants results in a markedly increased transepidermal water loss compared to a term infant.

B The skin in newborn infants is called the vernix caseosa.

C Epidermolysis bullosa may result in fusion of the fingers and toes and contractures of the limbs.

D Large congenital pigmented hairy naevi predispose to malignant melanoma.

E Repeated episodes of sunburn is a risk factor for malignant melanoma.

2. *These lesions (Fig. 22.1) were noted in a three-day-old infant. What is the most likely cause?*

3. *What is the diagnosis of the rash in Fig. 22.2?*

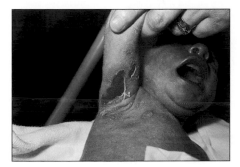

Fig. 22.1

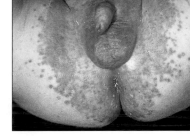

Fig. 22.2

4. *Which of the following rashes in childhood are itchy?*

A Varicella

B Scabies

C Molluscum contagiosum

D Seborrhoeic dermatitis

E Atopic eczema

5. *Which of the following statements about atopic eczema are true or false:*

A Onset is usually in the first month of life

B There is a strong association with asthma and hayfever

C Exacerbation may be caused by contact with peanuts

D In infants, involvement of the face is characteristic

E Cold sores in adults are a potential source of serious infection

1.

A True ❑ False ❑
B True ❑ False ❑
C True ❑ False ❑
D True ❑ False ❑
E True ❑ False ❑

2.

3.

4.

A True ❑ False ❑
B True ❑ False ❑
C True ❑ False ❑
D True ❑ False ❑
E True ❑ False ❑

5.

A True ❑ False ❑
B True ❑ False ❑
C True ❑ False ❑
D True ❑ False ❑
E True ❑ False ❑

6.

i) What is the most likely diagnosis of the rash shown in Fig. 22.3?

ii) What advice should this child's parents be given regarding clothing?

iii) What two pieces of advice should be given about bathing?

iv) What is the mainstay of topical treatment?

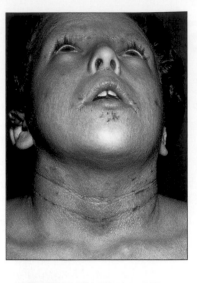

Fig. 22.3

7. *What is the cause of the lesions shown in Fig. 22.4?*

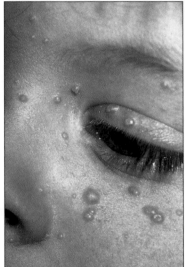

Fig. 22.4

8.

i) What is the cause of the lesion in Fig. 22.5?

ii) How can the diagnosis be confirmed?

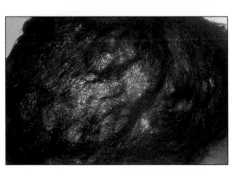

Fig. 22.5

6. i)

   ii)

   iii)

   iv)

7.

8. i)

   ii)

9. i)

9.

i) What is the cause of the itchy rash shown in Fig. 22.6?

ii) Which members of the family require treatment?

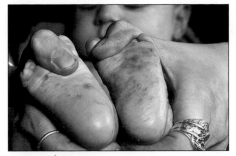

Fig. 22.6

10. *What is the most likely cause of the skin lesion shown in Fig. 22.7?*

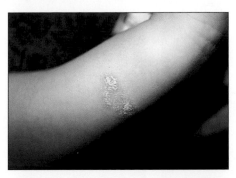

Fig. 22.7

11. *This 16-year-old boy has severe acne (Fig. 22.8).*

List two forms of drug therapy which may be helpful in treating this condition:

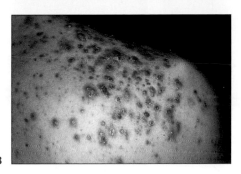

Fig. 22.8

ii)

10.

11.

12. Match the photographs with the case history by placing a tick in the corresponding box

Case history	Fig. 22.9			
	A	B	C	D
i) This child has had a daily spike of fever for two weeks				
ii) This child has hypertension				
iii) This child has haematuria				
iv) This child has been on cotrimoxazole for prophylaxis against pneumocystis infection				

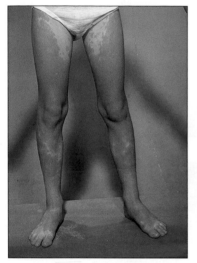

Fig. 22.9A

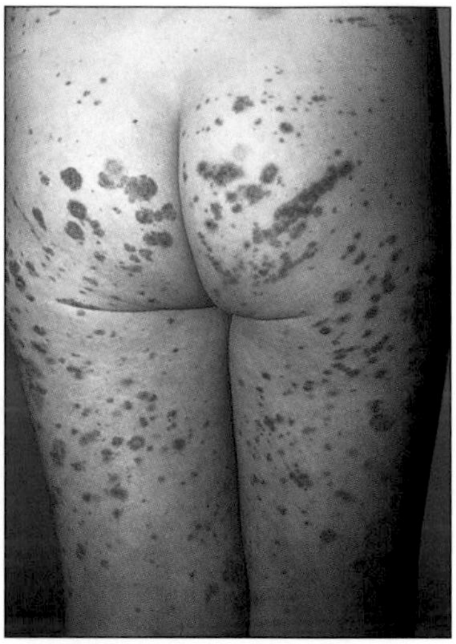

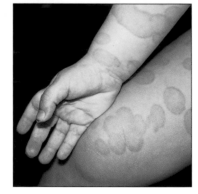

Fig. 22.9B

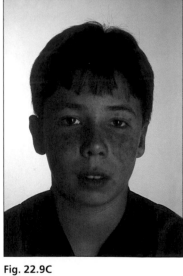

Fig. 22.9C

Fig. 22.9D

1. **A** *True.*
   B *False.* The vernix caseosa is the transient greasy film covering the skin in newborn term infants.
   C *True.* This may result from repeated blistering and healing in severe forms of this disorder.
   D *True.*
   E *True.*

2. *Staphylococcus aureus* infection causing bullous impetigo.

3. Candida napkin rash. In this condition the flexures are involved and there are satellite lesions; in irritant dermatitis the flexures are spared.

4. **A** *True.*
   B *True.*
   C *False.*
   D *False.*
   E *True.*

5. **A** *False.* It usually starts in infancy, but after two months of age.
   B *True.* Up to half the children with atopic eczema will develop asthma and/or hay fever.
   C *True.*
   D *True.*
   E *True.* May result in widespread herpes simplex infection (eczema herpeticum).

6. i) Atopic eczema.
   ii) To use loose pure cotton where possible, avoid nylon and pure woollen garments.
   iii) Avoid soap and biological detergents
       Use an emollient bath oil or an emulsifying ointment
       Pat rather than rub skin dry.
   iv) Emollients to moisturise the skin.

7. A pox virus causing molluscum contagiosum.

8. i) A ringworm fungus.
   ii) May fluoresce green/yellow under a special ultraviolet light (Woods light)
       Fungal hyphae seen on direct microscopy of skin scrapings
       Identification on fungal culture

9. i) Scabies.
   ii) The whole family should be treated whether or not they have evidence of infestation.

10. Psoriasis.

11. Keratolytic agents, e.g. benzoyl peroxide
    Topical antibiotics
    Topical retinoids
    Long-term oral antibiotic therapy
    Oral retinoids if unresponsive and severe.

Fig. 22.9

12. Case history	A	B	C	D
i) This child has had a daily spike of fever for two weeks	✓			
ii) This child has hypertension			✓	
iii) This child has haematuria, abdominal and joint pain		✓		
iv) This child has been on cotrimoxazole for prophylaxis against pneumocystis infection				✓

23 Endocrine and metabolic disorders

1. *Which of the following statements about type I diabetes mellitus in childhood are true or false:*

   A In the UK, the incidence is falling

   B There is autoimmune pancreatic β-cell damage

   C Weight gain is a recognised presentation

   D The diagnosis should be confirmed with a glucose tolerance test

   E Most children can be managed with oral hypoglycaemic agents and dietary modification

2. *James, aged 11, with type I diabetes mellitus, suddenly feels faint while playing football during the mid-morning break at school. His classmates call the teacher who finds him lying unresponsive in the playground. On arrival at the Accident and Emergency department his airway, breathing and circulation are satisfactory, but he is confused.*

   i) Which one of the following would you do immediately?

      A Measure urinary ketones

      B Give intravenous saline

      C Give intravenous insulin

      D Measure blood glucose at the bedside

      E Give intravenous antibiotics

   ii) Which of the following might have caused this episode? More than one answer may be true.

      A He played as a forward instead of his usual position in goal

      B He got up too late to have breakfast

      C He has a respiratory tract infection

      D He failed to take his usual mid-morning snack

      E He omitted his morning dose of insulin

3. *Which of the following are features of diabetic ketoacidosis:*

   A Weight loss

   B Abdominal pain

   C Sudden loss of consciousness

   D Slow, deep respiration

   E A normal blood glucose

1.

A	True ❏	False ❏
B	True ❏	False ❏
C	True ❏	False ❏
D	True ❏	False ❏
E	True ❏	False ❏

2. i) **A B C D E**

ii)

A	True ❏	False ❏
B	True ❏	False ❏
C	True ❏	False ❏
D	True ❏	False ❏
E	True ❏	False ❏

3.

A	True ❏	False ❏
B	True ❏	False ❏
C	True ❏	False ❏
D	True ❏	False ❏
E	True ❏	False ❏

Date	Insulin injection			Before breakfast	2hrs after breakfast	Before mid-day meal	2hrs after mid-day meal	Before evening meal	2hrs after evening meal	Before bed	During night	Comments
21/9						4						
22/9								4				
23/9						8						
24/9					5							
25/9												Visiting nan
26/9				5								
27/9									4			
28/9					4							
29/9				8								
30/9							10					
1/10									4			
2/10												Visiting nan
3/10							4					
4/10								3				
5/10							9					
6/10									8			
7/10					6							
8/10					4							
9/10							4					
10/10										6		
11/10										7		
12/10					5							

Please refer to your Doctor or Diabetes Nurse specialist as to when you should perform your tests.

Fig. 23.1

4. *Catherine, aged 15 years, has had type I diabetes mellitus for 7 years. Her insulin regimen has remained unchanged for the last 7 months. Her HbA$_{1C}$ has increased from 7.5% to 10.3% (normal range 3–6%). The most recent blood glucose levels as recorded in her book are shown Fig. 23.1. Select the single most likely explanation for these findings.*

4. A   B   C   D   E

A During the summer holidays she took less exercise

B She is taking less insulin to try to lose weight

C Some of the blood glucose measurements recorded are fictitious

D She is taking more insulin than she needs

E She is regularly drinking alcohol and eating snacks at parties

5. *Julie, aged seven, has diabetes mellitus. She developed a mild fever, sore throat and decreased appetite. Her blood glucose measurement read 'high'. She was unable to go to school and spent the day watching television. Although she was not eating, her parents maintained her usual insulin dose. The following afternoon she started to vomit and was admitted to hospital. On examination she has a temperature of 37.5°C and tonsillitis. Her pulse is 150/min, blood pressure 80/45. She is lethargic but able to talk coherently.*

5. i)

i) What two investigations would you perform to confirm that she has diabetic ketoacidosis?

ii) Select your first step in her management:

   A IV antibiotics

   B IV insulin

   C IV 0.9% saline

   D IV dextrose / saline

   E IV sodium bicarbonate

iii) List two potential complications associated with treating diabetic ketoacidosis:

iv) How might this episode have been prevented?

6. *Which of the following statements about hypoglycaemia are true or false:*

A It should be excluded in all critically ill children during resuscitation

B It is a recognised feature of alcohol poisoning

C Treatment with glucagon should be avoided

D It is a complication of steroid therapy

E It is associated with adrenal insufficiency

7. *Fig. 23.2 is a picture of Alina from Kosovo, aged two months, who is feeding poorly, is very lethargic and has severe constipation. Hypothyroidism is suspected.*

   i) List three physical signs which would support this diagnosis.

   ii) What is the commonest cause worldwide?

   iii) Why is this clinical picture rarely seen in the UK?

   Fig. 23.3 shows Alina following five months of therapy.

   iv) How long should the treatment be continued?

ii) A B C D E

iii)

iv)

6.

A True ❏ False ❏

B True ❏ False ❏

C True ❏ False ❏

D True ❏ False ❏

E True ❏ False ❏

7. i)

ii)

iii)

iv)

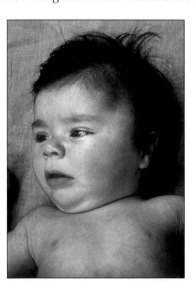

Fig. 23.2

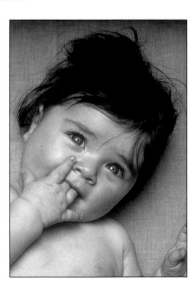

Fig. 23.3

8. *Hermione, aged 15 years, has had three months of diarrhoea, weight loss and palpitations (Fig. 23.4). You suspect hyperthyroidism.*

i) List three physical signs that would support your diagnosis.

ii) How would you confirm the diagnosis?

iii) What is the most likely pathophysiology?

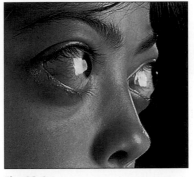

Fig. 23.4

8. i)

ii)

iii)

9. *Jenny is on long-term systemic steroid therapy.*

i) What side effect is shown in Fig. 23.5?

ii) List three other side effects:

iii) Give two ways in which they may be minimised.

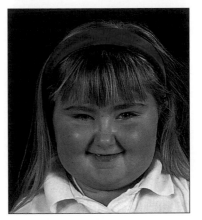

Fig. 23.5

9. i)

ii)

iii)

10. *Which of the following statements about phenylketonuria are true or false:*

A There is a deficiency of phenylalanine hydroxylase

B Screening is performed on day 1 of life

C There is an associated defect in skin pigmentation

D Treatment is with a low protein diet

E Poor control during pregnancy is associated with fetal abnormality

10.

A True ❑ False ❑

B True ❑ False ❑

C True ❑ False ❑

D True ❑ False ❑

E True ❑ False ❑

11. *Which of the following statements about inborn errors of metabolism are true or false?*

A At presentation in the neonatal period, a metabolic alkalosis is the commonest acid–base disturbance

B Albinism is associated with visual impairment

C Coma during a viral infection is characteristic of urea cycle defects

D Galactosaemia does not present until the infant is weaned

E Glycogen storage disorders are associated with hepatomegaly and hypoglycaemia

11.

A True ❑ False ❑

B True ❑ False ❑

C True ❑ False ❑

D True ❑ False ❑

E True ❑ False ❑

1. A *False.* In the UK the incidence is increasing and now affects 2 per 1000 children under 16 years of age.
    B *True.*
    C *False.* Weight loss is common at presentation.
    D *False.* The diagnosis is usually clear from the characteristic symptoms at presentation, together with a markedly raised plasma glucose and glycosuria.
    E *False.* Almost all children require insulin.

2. i) **D.** This presentation is suggestive of hypoglycaemia (a 'hypo').
    ii) **A.** *True.* Exercise more vigorous than usual may result in hypoglycaemia.
    B *True.*
    C *False.* This would be likely to cause hyperglycaemia.
    D *True.*
    E *False.* This would cause hyperglycaemia.

3. A *True.* Hyperglycaemia induces an osmotic diuresis leading to dehydration. Also, with insulin deficiency, the body becomes catabolic.
    B *True.*
    C *False.* This is associated with hypoglycaemia.
    D *True.* Kussmaul breathing is due to acidosis.
    E *False.* In children, the blood glucose is usually very high.

4. **C.** This is the most likely explanation for the discrepancy between the strikingly normal blood glucose recordings and the high HbA_{1C}. Taking less exercise, reducing the insulin dose or regularly drinking alcohol and eating snacks would result in high blood glucose levels. Taking more insulin than she needs would result in low blood glucose levels and normal HbA_{1C}.

5. i) Measure the blood glucose. It is usually >15 mmol/l
        Confirm that glucose and ketones are present in the urine
        Metabolic acidosis on blood gas analysis.
    ii) **C.** Her shock should be treated urgently. She will also require intravenous insulin and antibiotics, but these are not the first priority.
    iii) Hypoglycaemia. This is due to excess insulin administration.
        Hypokalaemia. This is because the insulin drives potassium into cells. It may cause arrythmias.
        Cerebral oedema. This may occur with rehydration.
        Aspiration from vomiting. This occurs from gastric dilatation and can be prevented by inserting a nasogastric tube.
    iv) Her insulin should have been increased to match her high blood glucose measurements.

6. A *True.*
    B *True.*
    C *False.* Intramuscular glucagon may be life saving prior to gaining intravenous access.
    D *False.* Steroid therapy is associated with hyperglycaemia.
    E *True.*

7. i) Pale, cold mottled dry skin
        Coarse facies
        Large tongue
        Umbilical hernia
        Hypotonia
        Delayed development
        Prolonged jaundice
        Goitre (occasionally).
    ii) Maternal iodine deficiency.
    iii) All newborn infants in the UK are screened for congenital hypothyroidism.
    iv) Lifelong.

8. i) Tremor
Tachycardia
Warm, vasodilated peripheries
Goitre (bruit)
Eye signs – exomphalos, ophthalmoplegia, lid retraction, lid lag
Rapid growth in height
Brisk reflexes
Psychosis.

ii) Measurement of serum TSH and free T_4. The TSH is very low and the free T_4 is raised.

iii) Auto-antibodies stimulating the thyroid gland.

9. i) Facial obesity, red cheeks characteristic of Cushingoid appearance.

ii) Short stature
Truncal obesity
Striae
Hirsutism
Hypertension
Immunosuppression
Glucose intolerance
Bruising, muscle wasting, osteoporosis, cataracts, psychological problems.

iii) Use lowest possible dose for shortest possible time
Topical administration, e.g. inhaled, cutaneous
Give on alternate days
Steroid sparing drugs.

10. A *True.*
B *False.* It is performed on day 5–7 when milk feeding has been established.
C *True.* This is the cause of the blue-eyed, blond hair phenotype.
D *False.* Treatment is with specific dietary phenylalanine restriction.
E *True.*

11. A *False.* The commonest acid–base disturbance is a metabolic acidosis.
B *True.*
C *True.*
D *False.* It presents in early infancy as galactose is present in both breast and formula milk.
E *True.*

24 Bones and joints

1. *Which of the following are variants of normal posture:*
   A   Bowing of the legs in an 18-month-old child
   B   Knock knees in a three-year-old child
   C   Persistent toe-walking in an 18-month-old child
   D   A toddler with flat feet
   E   A newborn infant's foot which is inverted but can be partially returned to a neutral position

2. *The parents of Suliman, aged 18 months, are concerned because he has suddenly stopped walking. On examination he is miserable but apyrexial. His left thigh is swollen. There is no discoloration of the skin and it is not warm to touch. He prefers to keep his left leg still but withdraws it on tickling his foot.*

   Select the most likely diagnosis:
   A   Osteomyelitis
   B   Septic arthritis
   C   Cellulitis
   D   Fractured femur
   E   Osteosarcoma

3. *Which of these statements about developmental dysplasia of the hip (congenital dislocation of the hip) are true or false:*
   A   The risk is increased following a ventouse delivery
   B   The risk is increased in a child with talipes equinovarus
   C   If clinically suspected at the newborn screening examination, an X-ray should be performed
   D   At 11 months of age, the Barlow and Ortolani manoeuvres are used for clinical detection
   E   The initial treatment is surgical

4. *Emma, aged 3½ years, starts to limp and complains of pain in her right thigh. There is no history of trauma but she has had a cold a few weeks ago. She is febrile and her pulse is 90/min. The most likely diagnoses are transient synovitis (irritable hip) and septic arthritis. Please tick in the table of clinical features and investigations shown below to demonstrate how the conditions may be differentiated. Some may apply to both conditions.*

	Transient synovitis (irritable hip)	Septic arthritis
High fever		
Systemically ill		
Marked pain on movement		
High acute phase reactant		
Hip effusion in ultrasound		

1.
A   True ☐   False ☐
B   True ☐   False ☐
C   True ☐   False ☐
D   True ☐   False ☐
E   True ☐   False ☐

2.   A   B   C   D   E

3.
A   True ☐   False ☐
B   True ☐   False ☐
C   True ☐   False ☐
D   True ☐   False ☐
E   True ☐   False ☐

4.

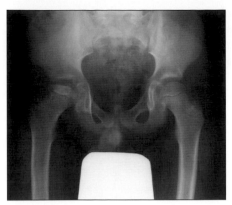

Fig. 24.1

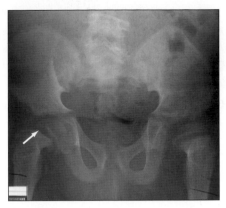

Fig. 24.2

5. *Match the following histories with the appropriate X-ray and give the diagnosis.*

A *An 8-year-old boy who presents with a few days of pain in the hip. On examination he looks well but is limping.*

B *An overweight 14-year-old girl with a one-day history of knee pain and limp.*

Case history	X-ray	Diagnosis
A	Fig. 24.1 or 24.2	
B	Fig. 24.1 or 24.2	

6. *Which of the following statements about disorders of the back are true or false:*

A It is rare to identify a cause for backache in children

B If associated with acute urinary problems, back pain is a neurosurgical emergency

C Abdominal pain is a recognised presentation

D Clinical assessment of scoliosis is best performed with the child standing upright

E Kyphosis is a cause of obstructive lung disease

6.

A True ❏ False ❏
B True ❏ False ❏
C True ❏ False ❏
D True ❏ False ❏
E True ❏ False ❏

7. *Which of the following statements about osteomyelitis are true or false:*

A Children with sickle cell anaemia are at increased risk

B Apparent paralysis of a limb is a recognised presentation

C The commonest pathogen in children is *Staphylococcus aureus*

D At presentation, subperiosteal new bone formation is identifiable on X-ray

E Direct spread through the epiphyseal growth plate into the joint occurs in infants

7.

A True ❏ False ❏
B True ❏ False ❏
C True ❏ False ❏
D True ❏ False ❏
E True ❏ False ❏

8. *Edward, aged three years, woke up complaining of pain in his right leg. During the day he refused to play in the garden with his older brother, preferring to watch television. On examination he is febrile at 39°C. His right knee is red and swollen and he cries if it is moved. There is a small healing insect bite on his right ankle.*

i) What is the most likely diagnosis?

ii) How would you confirm the diagnosis?

8. i)

ii)

9. *Karen, aged five years, has been unwell for six weeks with lethargy, fever and painful wrists and knees. On examination she has a temperature of 38.5°C and a subtle erythematous rash on her trunk. Her wrists are swollen, warm and painful to move. She has some cervical lymphadenopathy and her spleen is just palpable.*

Investigations reveal:

Hb 10 g/dl, WBC $14 \times 10^9/l$, neutrophils $7 \times 10^9/l$, platelets $366 \times 10^9/l$
Blood film normal, no atypical lymphocytes
ESR 70
ANA (Anti-nuclear antibody) –ve
Double stranded DNA –ve
ASO titre normal

Select the most likely diagnosis from the following:

A Acute lymphatic leukaemia

B SLE (systemic lupus erythematosis)

C EBV infection

D Post-streptococcal arthritis

E Juvenile idiopathic arthritis (juvenile chronic arthritis)

9. A B C D E

10. *Which of these statements about juvenile idiopathic arthritis (juvenile chronic arthritis) are true or false?*

A Fever, weight loss, rash and lymphadenopathy but no arthritis is a recognised presentation

B A positive rheumatoid factor is required to make this diagnosis

C Affected children are at increased risk of chronic anterior uveitis

D Non-steroidal anti-inflammatory drugs are used to treat pain

E A combination of splinting and active/passive physiotherapy is used to minimise joint deformity

10.

A True ❏ False ❏
B True ❏ False ❏
C True ❏ False ❏
D True ❏ False ❏
E True ❏ False ❏

11. *Jacob, aged 14 years, is concerned about his marked pectus excavatum (Fig. 24.3). On examination he is 190 cm tall (6′3″). He has long fingers, a high arched palate and wears glasses. The heart sounds are normal but there is a soft diastolic murmur at the left sternal edge.*

i) What is the most likely cause of his murmur?

ii) What condition does he have?

11. i)

    ii)

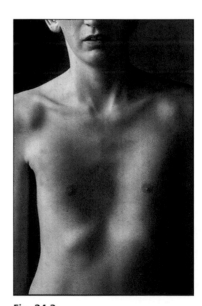

Fig. 24.3

1. A   *True.* This usually resolves by three years of age. Severe bowing, however, requires further investigation.
    B   *True.* This is common between two and seven years of age.
    C   *False.* Many children toe-walk intermittently, but not persistently.
    D   *True.*
    E   *False.* This is a feature of true talipes equinovarus. If the foot is inverted but can be manipulated to a neutral position it is a positional talipes, a variant of normal.

2. D. This may be accidental but non-accidental injury (NAI) needs to be considered in all unexplained fractures.

    In osteomyelitis and septic arthritis he would be unwell with a fever, the left thigh would be warm and discoloured and he would be unwilling to move the limb at all.
    Osteosarcoma would be extremely unusual at this age.

3. A   *False.* The risk is increased following breech delivery.
    B   *True.*
    C   *False.* An X-ray is unhelpful at this stage as the femoral head is radiolucent. An ultrasound is the investigation of choice.
    D   *False.* These manoeuvres are used at neonatal screening and at 6–8 weeks. Thereafter the clinical signs are asymmetrical thigh skin creases, limitation of hip abduction and shortening of the leg.
    E   *False.* Initial treatment is splinting the hips in abduction.

4. i)

	Transient synovitis (irritable hip)	Septic arthritis
High fever		✓
Systemically ill		✓
Marked pain on movement		✓
High acute phase reactant		✓
Hip effusion in ultrasound	✓	✓

5.

Case history	X-ray	Diagnosis
A	Fig. 24.1	Perthes disease
B	Fig. 24.2	Slipped femoral epiphysis

6. A   *False.* Backache in children is uncommon and requires thorough assessment.
    B   *True.* Acute urinary problems suggest spinal cord compression.
    C   *True.*
    D   *False.* A scoliosis is accentuated by the child bending forward.
    E   *False.* It can cause restrictive lung disease.

7. A   *True.*
    B   *True.*
    C   *True.*
    D   *False.* The only abnormality at presentation of acute osteomyelitis is soft tissue swelling.
    E   *True.* This can occur in infants as the growth plate is immature.

8. i)   Septic arthritis
    ii) Examination and culture of fluid aspirated from the knee joint.

9. E – juvenile idiopathic arthritis.
    Acute lymphatic leukaemia (ALL) is unlikely as the blood film is normal.
    SLE may have similar clinical features but is unlikely as the ANA and double stranded DNA are negative.
    Epstein–Barr virus (EBV) is unlikely as the blood film is normal and rarely causes widespread arthritis
    Post-streptococcal arthritis is unlikely as the ASO titre is normal.

10. A *True.* Especially in young children (Still's disease).
   B *False.* It is only positive in a minority of cases.
   C *True.* Especially the pauci-articular form.
   D *True.*
   E *True.*

11. i)   Aortic incompetence.
   ii) Marfan's syndrome

25 Neurological disorders

1. *The grandmother of Timothy, aged six months, is concerned because of his poor feeding and vomiting. On examination, his fontanelle is found to be bulging.*

i) What is the significance of this finding?

ii) List two possible causes.

2. *Julia, aged 10 years, has been suffering from headaches for three months. They occur 3–4 times per week and are interfering with her schooling. The headaches are generalised but not accompanied by visual disturbance and settle with an hour's bedrest. Her uncle died recently of a brain tumour and there is concern in the family that Julia has the same condition.*

i) What two further questions would help to exclude a brain tumour?

ii) Her eye, face and neck movements and neurological examination of her limbs are normal. List two other clinical features you would check to exclude a brain tumour.

3. *Christopher, aged 15 months, had been unwell with a runny nose and cough for a day. Suddenly, he became stiff, his eyes rolled upwards and both his arms and legs started shaking for two minutes. When examined two hours later he had recovered fully. A febrile convulsion is suspected.*

i) What three questions would you ask to support this diagnosis?

ii) Is an EEG indicated in this child?

iii) Are anti-convulsants indicated?

iv) What advice would you give his parents to prevent further febrile convulsions?

4. *Match the case history accompanied by an EEG, with the most likely diagnosis from the list provided.*

Case 1

David, a healthy 10-year-old has had an episode at school where he appeared to be in a trance, during which he was repetitively fidgeting with his hands. The attack lasted two minutes after which he complained of tiredness and then fell asleep (Fig. 25.1).

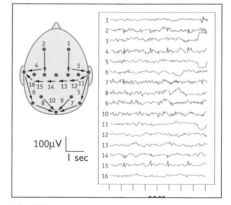

Fig. 25.1

1. i)

   ii)

2. i)

   ii)

3. i)

   ii) Yes ❑ No ❑
   iii) Yes ❑ No ❑
   iv)

4.

   Diagnosis

   Case 1 **A B C D E**

Case 2

Courtney, aged three years, has been noted to have episodes where she stops playing for a few seconds, stares blankly ahead before resuming her game. This happens several times a day (Fig. 25.2).

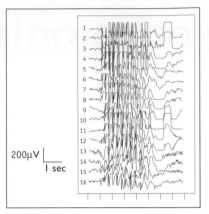

200μV | | sec

Fig. 25.2

Case 2   A B C D E

Case 3

Peter aged three months starts to have episodes during which he suddenly throws his head and arms forward. These occur in repetitive bursts. It was thought that they were due to colic but his mother is asking for reassurance that they are harmless (Fig. 25.3).

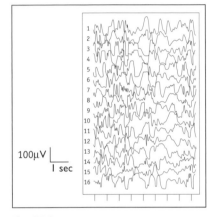

100μV | | sec

Fig. 25.3

Case 3   A B C D E

List of diagnoses:

A Temporal lobe epilepsy

B Generalised tonic clonic epilepsy

C Absence epilepsy (petit mal)

D Infantile spasms

E Benign Rolandic epilepsy

5. *Which of the following statements about cerebral palsy are true or false:*

A It is most commonly due to birth asphyxia.

B It is primarily a disorder of cognitive function.

C Feeding difficulties and persistent clenched fist are early clinical features.

D Hand preference in a child of 18 months is likely to be due to hemiparesis.

E Clinical signs evolve as the child grows older.

5.

A True ❑ False ❑

B True ❑ False ❑

C True ❑ False ❑

D True ❑ False ❑

E True ❑ False ❑

6. *Match the correct terminology about cerebral palsy with the description of the signs to complete the table below. Place a tick in the appropriate box.*

1   Poor tone, balance and delayed motor development in infancy; later inco-ordinate movements and intention tremor

2   All limbs affected but legs more than arms

3   Unilateral arm and leg involvement

4   Poor truncal tone and all four limbs affected to a similar degree

5   Fluctuating muscle tone with involuntary movements, e.g. athetosis (writhing)

	1	2	3	4	5
A Hemiplegia					
B Diplegia					
C Quadriplegia					
D Dyskinesia					
E Ataxia					

6.

7. *List two reasons why the number of infants born with neural tube defects (anencephaly and spina bifida) has declined markedly over the last 20 years:*

7.

8.

i) What is the lesion shown in Fig. 25.4?

ii) List two neurological problems this baby may have.

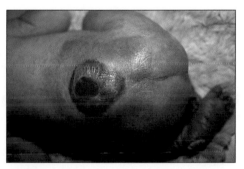

Fig. 25.4

8. i)

ii)

9. *The child shown in Fig. 25.5 has a large head.*

i) What sign is demonstrated?

ii) List two other clinical signs that would suggest hydrocephalus.

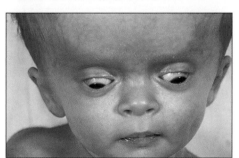

Fig. 25.5

9. i)

ii)

10.

i) What abnormality is shown shown in Fig. 25.6?

ii) With which disorder is this usually associated?

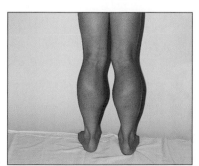

Fig. 25.6

10. i)

ii)

11. *Which of these statements about Duchenne's muscular dystrophy are true or false:*

A   The genetic defect is on chromosome 7

B   The absence of a family history makes the diagnosis unlikely

C   There is an abnormality of dystrophin

D   A positive Gower's sign is a recognised feature

E   The average age of onset is 12 years old

11.

A   True ❑   False ❑

B   True ❑   False ❑

C   True ❑   False ❑

D   True ❑   False ❑

E   True ❑   False ❑

12. *Stacey, aged two years, has been unsteady on her feet for a day, having had diarrhoea during the previous week. On examination she is afebrile with reduced muscle power and tone and no tendon reflexes can be elicited in her lower limbs. Six hours later she is unable to stand and the tendon reflexes in her upper limbs are now absent.*

i)   What is the most likely diagnosis?

ii) What is the most serious complication of this disorder?

12. i)

ii)

13.

i)   What is myotonia?

ii) How can it be demonstrated on physical examination?

13. i)

ii)

14. *What is the diagnosis of Fig. 25.7?*

14.

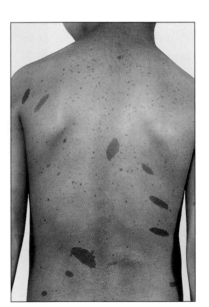

Fig. 25.7

1. i) Raised intracranial pressure.
   ii) Hydrocephalus
       Meningitis
       Space occupying lesion, e.g. subdural haematoma, tumour
       Cerebral oedema, e.g. post trauma

2. i) Is the headache worse on lying down?
       Does she have early morning vomiting?
       Has she had any personality or behaviour changes?
   ii) Fundi for papilloedema
       Visual fields (e.g. craniopharyngioma)
       Check height for growth failure (e.g. craniopharyngioma)

3. i) Did he have a fever before the convulsion?
       Has he had a previous febrile convulsion?
       Is there a family history of febrile convulsion?
       Is his development normal?
   ii) No.
   iii) No.
   iv) Keep cool by removing extra clothing.
       Give anti-pyretics as soon as he appears to be unwell.

4.

Case history	Diagnosis	EEG abnormality
Case 1	**A** Temporal lobe epilepsy	Focus in temporal lobe
Case 2	**C** Absence epilepsy (petit mal)	3 per second spike and wave
Case 3	**D** Infantile spasms	Hypsarrhythmia

5. **A** *False.* The cause is usually antenatal and of uncertain origin.
   B *False.* It is a motor disorder. Intellect can be normal although many have learning, visual, hearing or speech and language impairment.
   C *True.*
   D *False.* Beyond 12 months of age it is normal to start developing handedness.
   E *True.* The clinical signs evolve with age although the lesion itself is non-progressive.

6.

	1	2	3	4	5
Hemiplegia			✓		
Diplegia		✓			
Quadriplegia				✓	
Dyskinesia					✓
Ataxia	✓				

7. Natural decrease. This is possibly because of improved maternal nutrition.

   Antenatal screening: antenatal ultrasound and serum α-fetoprotein with option of termination of pregnancy if positive.

   Maternal folic acid supplementation.

8. i) Myelomeningocoele.
   ii) Paralysis of the legs
       Sensory loss in the legs
       Neuropathic bladder and bowel
       Hydrocephalus (from the Arnold–Chiari malformation).

9. i)   Downward deviation of the eyes (setting sun sign).
    ii) Rapidly increasing head circumference
         Separation of cranial sutures
         Anterior fontanelle tense or bulging
         Cranial nerve palsies
         Congested scalp veins

10. i)   Hypertrophy of the calf muscles.
    ii) Duchenne's muscular dystrophy.

11. A   *False*. It is an X-linked recessive disorder.
    B   *False*. About one-third are new mutations.
    C   *True*.
    D   *True*.
    E   *False*. The onset is usually pre-school.

12. i)   Guillain–Barré syndrome (post-infectious polyneuropathy). The classic presentation is with ascending weakness.
    ii) Respiratory failure. She must be closely monitored for this.

13. i)   Delayed relaxation after sustained muscle contraction.
    ii) Inability to relax the grip after clenching of the fist, as in shaking hands.

14. Neurofibromatosis. These are café au lait spots.

26 The child with special needs

1. *Gemma was born by spontaneous vaginal delivery at term weighing 2.8 kg. At birth she was noted to have the clinical features of Down's syndrome. Antenatal screening had revealed a risk of 1 in 100 for this condition but her 28-year-old mother declined amniocentesis. The family are seen by the consultant paediatrician who confirms the diagnosis clinically and arranges to see both parents.*

   i) List four key topics that should be discussed with them.

   ii) Before discharge home list three health professionals who should be contacted.

2. *Pedro, a seven-year-old boy with spastic quadriplegia, moves into your general practice area. He is confined to a wheelchair and has attended a special school.*

   i) List five health professionals he is likely to need.

   ii) Complete the table giving one example of a common medical problem Pedro may encounter in each of the systems listed:

	Example of medical problem
Respiratory	
Gastrointestinal	
Urinary	
Cerebral	
Back	
Lower limbs	

3. *Simon presented at three years of age with delayed walking. He was diagnosed as having Duchenne's muscular dystrophy. By 15 years of age, although still attending mainstream school, he is confined to a wheelchair and requires mask ventilation at night because of poor respiratory effort. He presents to hospital with a severe chest infection, a rapidly increasing oxygen requirement and is developing respiratory failure.*

   Which of the following statements are true or false:

   A Artificial ventilation should not be considered as he has an incurable disease

   B He should be considered urgently for a lung transplant

   C He should not be informed about the seriousness of his illness even if he asks about it as it is likely to upset him

   D In the UK, should he not wish to be ventilated this must be adhered to as he fully understands the consequences

   E You should not consent to his and his parents' wishes to be discharged home for palliative care

---

1. i)

   ii)

2. i)

   ii)

3.

   A True ☐ False ☐

   B True ☐ False ☐

   C True ☐ False ☐

   D True ☐ False ☐

   E True ☐ False ☐

1. i) What the condition is
        Why it has occurred – genetic basis
        Need to confirm the diagnosis with chromosomal analysis
        Potential immediate medical problems (feeding difficulties, duodenal atresia, cardiac defects)
        Long-term problems (medical, developmental, educational and social problems)
        What to say to relatives and friends
        Self-help groups
        Written information
        Follow-up arrangements
    ii) General practitioner. This is to communicate the diagnosis and follow-up plans
        Health visitor and/or community paediatric nurses
        Child development service
        Social worker, if appropriate

2. i) Paediatrician
        Physiotherapist
        Occupational therapist
        Speech and language therapist
        Clinical psychologist
        Dietician
        Social worker
        Specialist health visitor/Community nurse

    ii)

	Example of medical problem
Respiratory	Recurrent chest infections, aspiration
Gastrointestinal	Gastro-oesophageal reflux, poor swallowing, poor nutrition, constipation, faecal incontinence
Urinary	Incontinence, urinary tract infections
Cerebral	Cognitive delay, epilepsy
Back	Scoliosis/kyphosis
Lower limbs	Muscle wasting, contractures, dislocation of the hips, fractures

3. A   *False.* Artificial ventilation for an acute deterioration should be considered as it might extend or provide good quality life.
    B   *False.* The underlying problem is progressive muscular weakness.
    C   *False.* Most children of his age will already know about their illness and its implications and should have the opportunity to discuss them.
    D   *False.* If he has an adequate understanding of his illness he is able to give and refuse consent. However legal precedent has only supported children's views to *accept* therapy, but not to refuse it when this is in conflict with the views of their parents or medical staff.
    E   *False.* As long as he and his parents are made aware that he is likely to die without ventilatory support their wishes should be respected. Palliative care should be provided at home.

Index